THE XO FACTOR

THE XO FACTOR

and how it can destroy your
arteries, your heart, your life!

the work of
Kurt A. Oster, M.D.
Donald J. Ross, Ph.D.

as told to
Hazel H. Richmond Dawkins

edited by
Nicholas Sampsidis
Michael D. Morrison

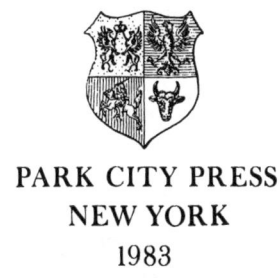

PARK CITY PRESS
NEW YORK
1983

First Edition

Printed in the United States of America

Library of Congress Catalog Card Number: 83-62282
ISBN: 0-943550-02-5

Book Design and Illustrations by Dimitry Schidlovsky
Cover Design by Tom Watson

This book is dedicated
to the memory of my parents

Regina and Benno

victims of the Nazi Holocaust
whose place of burial lies unmarked and unknown

−Kurt A. Oster

Publisher's Note

The medical information contained in this book is based on clinical research findings and on documented scientific evidence. The publication of this book does not, however, constitute the practice of medicine and is not intended as a substitute for the guidance of a personal physician who may be aware of specifics concerning an individual's health which may preclude one from applying the nutritional guidelines contained herein.

Acknowledgements

It's most satisfying to know you're working with material that has the potential to help people all over the world. *The XO Factor* has been a most rewarding project.

When I first read about the work of Kurt A. Oster and Donald J. Ross in the *Bridgeport Post* in 1981 I was impressed with the concept. I realized how many could benefit from the work – if only they knew about it. That was two years and four reams of typing paper ago.

The help and caring of all my family have been wonderful, particularly my husband Colin and Alexandra, my daughter. Without Sybil's shiatsu and Meb's sturdy shoulder in times of need, the work would have been that much harder and taken that much longer.

Suzanne Porter-Zadera, the librarian at Park City Hospital, has been an invaluable source of scientific and medical literature.

I am grateful to Linda Burke, Jill Kalen, and Dena Gechter for their assistance in compiling the manuscript.

Hazel Richmond Dawkins
July 1983

"The malignant influence of continuous homogenized milk intake containing biologically available xanthine oxidase, especially in youth, is in my opinion, a greater health evil than smoking cigarettes."

—Kurt A. Oster, M.D.

Preface

In the glut of books on nutrition, diet, and contaminant scares, the reader may ask, "Why another book?" Part of the justification lies in the confusion such a large mass of often unsubstantiated information has generated. On a popular television show, one woman listener, confused about a multitude of dietary taboos, asks, "What is there left which is allowed or healthy to eat or drink?" It seems obvious her question will not be adequately or honestly answered by the forces of vested interests and those devoted to maintenance of the status quo. Nowhere is this more evident than in the inertia surrounding the proposed dietary causes and treatment of atherosclerosis.

A widespread fixation on the bankrupt serum cholesterol risk factor theory and love affair with medical technology has created great resistance to new ideas and countertheories. In its stagnancy, the low cholesterol theory and its proponents continue to exercise control and repeatedly waste millions of scarce research dollars on such fiascos as the Multiple Risk Factor Intervention Trial (which cost the taxpayers $115,000,000 and, due to poor design and planning, proved nothing).

Part of the problem lies with the failure of the research community to recognize the potential causes of atherosclerosis, causes which manifest themselves in youth (as shown by the Korean War autopsy studies of Enos and his associates) and are related to the dietary components of this physically active, relatively stress-free time of life.

Another serious fallacy in the modern concept of atherosclerotic research is the tendency to view the disease in terms of isolated symptoms, most notably in the coronary arteries of the heart, rather than as a silent pathological process which can befall the entire vascular system. As long as the establishment does not occupy itself with the cause of atherosclerosis in each and every organ system of the body and as long as it confines itself to the narrow field of coronary artery disease, which may have multifactorial causes such as blood clots and spasms, the establishment will never succeed in elucidating even one cause.

This book confines itself to the question, "Which commonly consumed food in the western world may be causally connected with atherosclerosis in the young?" It is not concerned about the process of how the originally established lesion spreads and becomes life-threatening. This book does not deal with the quick-fix preoccupation of modern medicine. It has no drama of heart transplant, multiple bypass operations, transluminal balloon compression of lesions, and blood clot disintegration which makes good television propaganda and fills the columns of the media writers. Just the opposite...this book will deal with the prevention of an insidious process which will make all these drama-filled, gory and costly procedures eventually unnecessary. This may ultimately lead the way to the saving of billions of medical care cost dollars now frantically spent to save one life for an illness which might not have occurred in the first place. This book shows that 50 percent of atherosclerotic illnesses are man-made, poorly diagnosed, and mistakenly treated as isolated catastrophes.

The food accused in this book is cow's milk, a food which has been changed over the years by processing into an unrecognizable physicochemical emulsion which bears very little resemblance to the original, natural, and nutritional milk which is the main life-supporting material for growing calves. A basic difference between human and cow's milk is the content of an enzyme: namely, xanthine oxidase, or XO. Human milk contains only negligible amounts of this powerful oxidizing substance, whereas the amount in cow's milk is abundant.

This book is not against milk per se, but against the indiscriminate processing of a good food by those who have as their motives: profits, impeding scientific progress, and the need to cling to the old prejudicial slogan that cow's milk is the perfect food. It is therefore understandable that trade organizations, such as the National Dairy Council and their grantees, will combat the facts disclosed in this book, since these facts threaten to upset the milk cart and a very stable economic base.

What is not easy to comprehend is the attitude of the scientific fraternities toward the xanthine oxidase theory. Many researchers, whose grants and livelihoods depend on the unproven assumption that cholesterol is the causative agent of atherosclerotic lesions, simply ignore the xanthine oxidase concept and its attendant focus on the fat-carrying, life-sustaining phospholipids, especially plasmalogen. The monomaniacal preoccupation of the establishment with cholesterol, a substance the body utilizes in response to injury to the artery wall, has made it almost impossible to be heard in the scientific assembly. Because the xanthine oxidase theory runs counter to accepted beliefs, it has been met with silence and, if examined, with a few flawed scientific experiments financed by the National Dairy Council.

As some consolation, several undaunted researchers have, however, confirmed each and every one of our findings. Still the United States Food and Drug Administration, despite these confirmations, has not seen fit to examine the continued use and distribution of homogenized, pasteurized bovine milk, which, in our opinion, has been proven to a high degree of scientific accuracy to be a major culprit in the *causation* of atherosclerosis, a disease which starts in youth when the greatest consumption of this food takes place. How powerful is the influence of the Dairy Industry in relation to the health and well-being of the American people, the consumers who subsidize this industry to the tune of $2,000,000,000 a year?

In order to interest a larger audience which may show more objectivity and open-mindedness to the problem, this book is intended for the lay reader (and milk consumer). Hopefully, it will demonstrate to the concerned parents of youth the dangers of denatured, processed, pasteurized, homogenized bovine milk and the enzyme contained in it.

Objections continue to present themselves to our theory, particularly those clinging to the outdated belief that the size of the xanthine oxidase molecule is too large to penetrate the intestine and enter the bloodstream. This reminds me of the Maginot Line concept of the French Army who also thought that the Germans could not pass through, but they did. We have proven that the xanthine oxidase molecule can pass through the intestine in its homogenized form. We have proven that the enzyme can be found in tissues where it should never be. We have proven that the enzyme causes specific antibodies in milk-drinking persons. And we are trying to prove that a vitamin in large amounts — namely, folic acid — can prevent the progression of the injury which xanthine oxidase exerts on our vital tissues. Finally, we have also shown a way to prevent the entire pathological process from occurring merely by preventing the ingestion of the enzyme in cow's milk.

I want to thank Dr. Donald J. Ross for his untiring efforts to find xanthine oxidase in human tissues, to elucidate the liposome complex, and to help perfect the antibody determination in human serum. Likewise, Barbara O'Neill, R.N., for her untiring efforts and help in patient care in the difficult combination of research and nursing. I would also like to acknowledge the patience of my wife, who tolerated and abetted my all-encompassing time — and money-consuming research efforts, which together with an active medical practice made life quite hectic, stimulating, and often controversial. Finally, I want to thank Mrs. Hazel Richmond Dawkins, who first approached me with the idea of writing this book.

Kurt A. Oster, M.D.

Contents

Physician, Heal Thyself!

Dr. Kurt Oster's heart attack arrived with classic stealth. He mentally noted his "acute indigestion." He felt uncomfortable. Very uncomfortable.

"That dinner really upset me," he told his wife as they arrived at the party. He did not, at first, consider that the pain could be anything serious.

The hostess greeted them with a smile, but when she looked at Oster she frowned: "Do you feel all right? You look pale."

By the time he left the party, virtually every one had told Oster he looked dreadful. He knew something was wrong. Gradually, he realized his "acute indigestion" might have another name: heart attack.

Oster went to the hospital for a battery of tests to see if he'd had a heart attack. All the results were negative. He was then ordered to take a series of gastrointestinal tests since the radiating symptoms of a gastrointestinal disorder may mimic those of a heart attack. Still the results were negative.

As a last resort, Oster decided to seek a second opinion on his "acute indigestion." Perhaps the first tests to see if he'd had a heart attack had missed something. He consulted one of the leading cardiologists in the area. Again the results were negative.

"Nothing wrong with you," said the physician. "Back to work."

Then came the moment of truth.

Before he was to start hospital rounds on that Tuesday morning in August 1965, Nurse Barbara O'Neill, who was also his secretary, took yet one more electrocardiogram. The EKG, a tracing of the heart's electrical activities, shows any unusual changes.

Now, two weeks after his "acute indigestion," after numerous tests, changes in Oster's heart finally showed up. Oster had suffered a heart attack. The description was:

"An anterior myocardial infarction."

Apparently simple words describing a heart attack, words that in this case referred specifically to the death of part of the heart muscle at the front of the heart.

Worst of all, it had happened to him once before, nine years previously, although then the case record was different. Then it read, "An inferior myocardial infarction," for that attack had been at the rear of the heart.

The diagnosis of the first heart attack, like the second, was confirmed by changes in his electrocardiogram, by the measurement of blood enzymes released from the damaged heart muscle, and by the weakness he felt.

That first time, in 1956, as he lay in bed enduring the tedium of bedrest, slowly recovering, he had begun to plot the strategy of treatment that would help prevent a recurrence. After all, he was a heart specialist. He knew what he had to do, or thought he did. Doctors knew what to do, or thought they did.

For people who had specific symptoms, drugs were available. Oster's condition, however, did not mandate any. He was advised to follow a modest regimen of exercise and to keep his weight normal even though he wasn't overweight. He was reminded to reduce salt, fat, and, oh yes, cholesterol, while eating a balanced diet. But he already was eating a balanced diet! He had eliminated tobacco back in 1951 and, except for an occasional glass of wine, he wasn't a consumer of alcoholic beverages. Still, he was being advised to change his lifestyle. What was left to change he wondered? Perhaps he was overworking himself?

Skeptical as he was about the prescribed formula for recovery, Oster made a resolution while in the hospital in 1956. He would be extremely conscientious about lifestyle and dietary considerations.

"Why are you giving me eggs for breakfast?" he demanded of the nurse when his first breakfast arrived.

"Don't you like eggs?"

"I love them, but I must think of my serum cholesterol. I'm in the hospital because I've had a heart attack."

"Don't worry. This is your quota for last week," the nurse soothed.

The next morning, Oster was amazed to find his breakfast again consisted of two boiled eggs.

"More eggs?" he demanded.

"This week's quota," came the swift reply.

When the nurse again brought a tray with two boiled eggs for the third consecutive morning, Oster gave her a puzzled look.

"Next week's quota."

Furious, Oster picked up the eggs and hurled them against the door. He knew what the medical establishment said about preventing heart attacks.

Try to lower the cholesterol and fat in your diet.

Use polyunsaturates.

Change your way of eating, and change your way of life. Oster took these nutritional guidelines seriously. He inflicted the regimen — which was tedious and therefore sometimes miserable — not only on himself but on his family as well for nine years. But with the occurrence of the second heart attack, it was obvious this widely advocated strategy had not worked. It was in fact useless. Perhaps worse than useless, for one tended to become a dietary hypochondriac.

Kurt A. Oster, M.D., arrived in the United States in the late 1930s as a refugee from Hitler's Nazi Germany. An alumnus of two of Europe's most distinguished universities, Oster was a graduate of the Medical School of the University of Cologne and had the further asset of a graduate degree in chemistry from the University of Berlin. He had served as the Chief Resident in Pediatrics in a large hospital in Berlin.

He could compete in the New World.

Once he had completed the requisite AMA-approved hospital internship, his special and comparatively rare qualifications brought him a research fellowship almost immediately. The work was medical research, first with Mount Sinai Hospital in New York City, an institution of formidable reputation, then later with the College of Physicians and Surgeons at Columbia University.

At each of these New York institutions, he worked in collaboration with highly respected, world-renowned scientists. Included among these was Charles Lieb, one of the co-discoverers of prostaglandin precursors, secretions of the prostate gland.

Oster's work at Mount Sinai and Columbia formed the foundation for a growing reputation. He and his colleagues published more than half a dozen papers that made outstanding contributions to the international body of medical and biochemical literature.

During this time Oster made some crucial observations about human tissues and their chemical reactions. The observations were of significance because they would influence his subsequent work on cardiovascular disease. Years later Oster would be fond of quoting Louis Pasteur: "Fortune always favors the prepared mind." The priceless fund of scientific knowledge that Oster built up in the first years he worked in America was to have far-reaching consequences. It became the foundation for his quick understanding of the phenomenon he was to observe years later.

In 1940 Oster became certified as a Diplomate of the National Board of Medical Examiners, an extremely challenging certification for graduates of foreign universities because a mastery of the English language was a prerequisite for passing the examination.

The Japanese attack on Pearl Harbor in December 1941 brought another upheaval in Oster's life. Peacetime activities were laid aside as

America mobilized to fight history's second global war. Oster was abruptly snatched from academe. He joined McKesson and Robbins in Fairfield, Connecticut, in 1943. McKesson was one of the largest wholesale drug companies in America and continues to be so today. Oster was eventually to serve McKesson both as research pharmacologist and medical director for over three decades.

"My first project for McKesson," he recalls, "was a massive war-time program. It took second place in national importance and priority only to the Manhattan Project: the development of the a-tomic bomb. We were one of eighteen firms certi-fied by the U.S. government to produce a new drug called penicillin for the Armed Forces.

"Those were hectic years. Because of the cri-tical shortage of medical specialists, I took my Connecticut medical boards and went into private practice in internal medicine and cardiology. At first I could attend to my private practice only in the evenings, of course."

A hospital near his office also needed special-ists in internal medicine. Oster began an associa-tion with Bridgeport's Park City Hospital that eventually led to his becoming the Director of the Electrocardiographic Laboratory, Chief of the Sec-tion of Cardiology, and Chairman of the Depart-ment of Medicine. His talents were recognized by his peers.

For almost twenty years, Oster pursued this busy life, a success at many levels. A Fellow of both the American College of Physicians and the American College of Cardiology, as well as the American College of Clinical Pharmacology, and later the American College of Nutrition, he was also an active member of numerous scientific soci-eties and medical associations. He even found time to teach pharmacology at the University of

Bridgeport.

There was just one jarring note. During this time the healer, the eminent cardiologist, had two heart attacks.

The first he accepted.

The second confounded him. He had adhered strictly to the edicts of the medical establishment. Yet despite this, a second heart attack happened. It began to dawn upon Oster that the so-called heart specialists really didn't know the causes of heart and circulatory diseases and certainly didn't know how to prevent them. He could no longer afford to rely on the guidelines of his medical colleagues. How could anyone know if he would survive a third heart attack?

Once again, he lay in his sickbed, searching for an answer. He reviewed in his mind everything he knew about the heart, its functions and frailties, about treatments, about what he told his patients and, above all, he reviewed his research findings thus far.

Oster pondered the edicts that he had long taken on faith, edicts that he had accepted because they were part of common medical practice and were based on the testimony of reputable researchers. Too much of what the medical world accepted as truth about heart and circulatory diseases was, he realized, all too frequently based on the statistical study of such diseases in population groups, the branch of science known as epidemiology.

In the right context, epidemiology is a valuable tool in the control of a disease within a population, particularly those diseases which are transmitted by insects, as in malaria and typhus. However, the second heart attack dictated to Oster that the application of epidemiology to the control of heart and circulatory diseases had its limitations. In fact, epidemiology had become little more than a game played by the cardiologists, a game in which statistics and population groups had become the pawns, a game played with millions of cardiac patients and their families.

Epidemiology has another drawback. It is subject to considerable scientific error and, as more than one person has pointed out, statistics are only as reliable as the person who is trying to make a case out of them...and sometimes, not even that.

So now, after twenty years and two heart attacks, Kurt A. Oster, M.D., made a vital decision. He promised himself to adjust his workstyle, to cut down on his many commitments and to step up his lifelong interest in medical research. He would, he told himself, concentrate on research into atherosclerosis, the underlying cause of his two heart attacks, the disease behind so many serious health problems.

In Oster's mind it had become a case of: "Physician, heal thyself!"

A Medical Detective Story

If a person had a heart attack in the 1960s, chances were that the doctor would have warned him or her about the villain cholesterol and about those dangerous saturated fats in food. Cholesterol and saturated fats were generally accepted by the medical community as being the culprits which caused atherosclerosis and led to heart disease. Even in the 1980s, this still unproved notion has changed little.

Oster actually started his laboratory research into heart and circulatory disease several years before his second heart attack. It began with a thorough search of medical literature. When Oster looked into the existing library of reports on the subject, he was amazed to find an abundance of information, but nothing that actually proved the cholesterol-lipid theory in humans.

He simply could not find a single study – not one in the total body of decades of research – that added up to anything more about the role of cholesterol and saturated fats than "maybe, but not proved." Eventually, over the years, several studies even suggested that certain polyunsaturated oils, far from being the great, magic, cholesterol-reducing hope for which they had been promoted, might even be hazardous to one's health.

As Oster delved deeper into his investigation of the cholesterol theory, he found, incredibly, that whole industries had been established, millions of individual lifestyles changed, countless diet books propelled onto the nation's bestseller lists...all based on the most inconclusive statistical juggling. Special vested interest groups were exploiting an unproven hypothesis while making a mockery of the scientific method.

After twenty years of uncritical acceptance of one classic medical mind-set about the role of dietary fats and cholesterol in atherosclerosis, Oster needed time to redirect his thinking. If he dismissed cholesterol and saturated fats in the diet as one of the primary causes of atherosclerosis, as he now did, where did the real culprit lurk?

It was in the latter part of 1964 that Oster fully committed himself to finding a valid dietary cause of atherosclerosis. He began at ground zero and started with the most basic research. He started by closely scrutinizing and comparing the structure and biochemistry of healthy and diseased arterial tissue. And as with all medical research of this sort, Oster knew that he was embarking on a hunt. He was well-armed with intuition and years of experience, but he did not have any guarantee when, or even if, his search would flush the predator.

Practical matters had to be organized. Oster arranged to use the pathology laboratory at his home base, Park City Hospital. He needed the use of a micro-photographic camera and located one at a nearby Veterans Administration Hospital.

Then he recruited a team to help him. The hospital's pathologist, Peter Hope-Ross, was enlisted. Phillip Brown, a student who was supporting himself as a laboratory technician, also joined the project.

A grant to Oster from the Greater Bridgeport Chapter of the Connecticut Heart Association, of which he was a founding member, was passed on to Brown to pay for the student's yeoman services over the months ahead.

Oster's insight and his years of research experience helped guide him in his decision to begin the investigation by studying a fatty component of cell membranes known as plasmalogen. Although plasmalogen, which belongs to the phospholipid family, was known to be an essential part of many cell membranes its presence was generally not appreciated by the medical community in America.

In Germany, where Oster received his medical training, plasmalogen had been studied much more extensively.   Robert Feulgen, the German biochemist, discovered plasmalogen and is the father of plasmalogen research. Gertrude Debuch, another German biochemist, whom Oster visited in 1968, had also conducted extensive research into plasmalogen at the University of Cologne. Thus, Oster's fluency in the German language and his personal contacts put him in a favorable position in the race to uncover the biochemical secrets behind a possible cause of heart and circulatory disease. His personal contacts provided a source of information not open to most other researchers in the United States, although the work of the German biochemists had been published and the information was in the public domain.

Laying the Foundation

Surrounding each one of the cells which make up normal heart and artery wall tissue is a membrane described by the men of science as a phospholipid-cholesterol mosaic interspersed with protein. The membrane is responsible for a variety of important functions, including the transport of oxygen, ions, and nutrients to the interior of cells. Thirty percent of the phospholipid portion of the membrane in human heart muscle cells is composed of plasmalogen.

G. E. Ansell, a renowned English biochemist, described phospholipids as "ubiquitous components of membrane systems." J. L. Thudichum, the leading original researcher of phospholipids commented that phospholipids "...are the center, life, and chemical soul of all bioplasm whatsoever, that of plants as well as animals."

The presence of plasmalogen within the phospholipid component of the cell membrane is essential to the integrity of the cell membrane in much the same way that mortar is an ingredient vital to the cohesiveness of a brick wall. One can imagine what would happen to a brick wall if 30 percent of the mortar fell out.

It is astonishing that with all of the medical research done on cardiovascular tissue, little or no attention has been paid to plasmalogen, a major component of the cell membrane.

The phospholipid plasmalogen is widely scattered throughout the human body. It is in the human heart muscle and in artery walls. Plasmalogen is also present in the myelin sheath surrounding nerve fibers, in certain portions of the kidney, in the mucous membranes of the large intestine, and in the adrenal cortex, the outer layer of the small glands which rest on top of the kidney. However, plasmalogen is not found in other parts of the human anatomy. The most apparent locations where it cannot be found are the liver cells proper and some areas of the mucous membrane of the small intestine.

Because the phospholipid plasmalogen plays such a crucial role in the integrity of cell membranes, Oster was interested in establishing whether a relationship existed between atherosclerosis and plasmalogen. The biochemical composition of plasmalogen suggested to Oster's trained mind that it could be the weak link in the cell membrane with regard to atherosclerosis.

Thus, Oster resolved he would continue to investigate plasmalogen, as he had done previously in his career. Earlier he had established that the anatomical distribution of plasmalogen in rats was dependent upon sex hormones. This earlier work demonstrated that the kidneys of male rats have abundant plasmalogen, while those of female rats contain very little plasmalogen. To Oster, plasmalogen was an essential starting point.

Before Oster's work, the scientific journals showed that only a few teams of researchers had ever investigated the relationship between plasmalogen and heart disease. Most others were too preoccupied with establishing a connection between dietary cholesterol and saturated fats and diseases of the heart and arteries. Yet the theory that cholesterol and saturated fats in food causes these health problems is nothing more than an unproven hypothesis which, somehow, has been blindly followed by many researchers.

Some of the most prominent supporters of the cholesterol theory, those who would later hold top positions at the best funded research institutions in the United States, explained in 1967 that phospholipids did have a role in cardiovascular disease but a very minor one. An often quoted paper on the subject, "Fat Transport in Lipoproteins: An Integrated Approach to Mechanisms and Disorders," was written by D. S. Frederickson, R. T. Levy, and R. S. Lees. This paper, which appeared in the *New England Journal of Medicine*, theorized that the role of phospholipids in the blood serum was merely that of a "detergent." What were the scientific reasons for this conclusion given by the writers of the paper? Their scientific intuition. The leading "specialists" in the country on heart disease were guessing!

A Crack in the Edifice

It was just under two years before his second heart attack that Kurt A. Oster, M.D., actually began his research on plasmalogen, the slow measured groping in the dark that characterizes all basic, original research. With luck and a spot of divine inspiration, there might come that sudden spark of light.

Oster and his group took over the hospital's pathology lab after the technicians had left for the day, whenever surgical specimens or autopsy materials were available.

The basic work was on unfixed tissue from autopsies. The term unfixed indicates a tissue has not been soaked in formaldehyde, the standard procedure by which surgical specimens are preserved. Oster could not use autopsy material immersed in formaldehyde because the fuchsin sulfurous acid stain, used to define the presence of plasmalogen, reacts with the chemical group known as aldehydes. As its name suggests, formaldehyde is in the aldehyde family. Had Oster used tissues fixed in formaldehyde, he would have obtained false-positive results, and every tissue sample would have appeared to contain plasmalogen. So, tissues not fixed in formaldehyde were used. This in itself presented a specific problem. Because the tissues were not fixed, Oster and his team had to work quickly, before the tissues suffered cellular death.

First, Oster's team sectioned tissue block samples with the freezing microtome, a cutting tool used in histology. Then, with painstaking care, they mounted the wafer-thin tissue sections on slides for staining and observation. Analyzing the results, the most time-consuming step, took hours.

They worked long into the evening, most evenings, for after the slide work had been analyzed, the details of the observations had to be recorded. The scrupulous entry of procedures and results in a continuing record is basic to any research enterprise. The methodology is prescribed and unvarying so that the experiment can be repeated by interested parties anywhere in the world. The procedure provides the only acceptable basis for later reports to professional journals and scientific bodies.

Even when the note-taking was completed, one final step remained for the research team whenever some abnormalities were suspected. Phillip Brown, the technician, would rush the slides to the Veteran's Hospital and use their invaluable camera to take microphotographs. Without these photos, there would not have been any permanent evidence, no indisputable record. Any evidence that might have shown up on the laboratory slides which Oster was making would have faded and disappeared within a few hours due to the impermanent nature of the fuchsin sulfurous acid stain. A photo was absolutely essential.

As the weeks went by, the stack of notebooks

grew. The results that filled them were routine and unremarkable. The information gleaned was a large body of material, but none was new or even unexpected.

And so Oster continued, with the patience of the dedicated professional and the eagerness of the zealot.

Finally came the night in November 1964 when the perplexed scientist stood at the desk in an office adjacent to the laboratory looking at something that couldn't be.

"That's impossible!" he thought.

"Why would that tissue be different? How could it be different?"

A little while earlier he had observed Phillip Brown cutting and mounting the tissue. Tissues provided by the hospital should contain plasmalogen, that essential component of cell membranes. This one didn't.

After examining it through the microscope, Oster picked up the stained slide which lacked the purple color characteristic of plasmalogen and looked at it curiously. He held it up to the light, turned it over as though he were looking for an explanation on the back. He shook his head thoughtfully.

"It doesn't make sense. I've double checked all the preparations. It's all absolutely correct. Except...this." He shrugged. Phillip Brown, standing in the background, wondered anxiously if he'd done something wrong. Why else would Dr. Oster be so concerned?

"Let's go over the slides again, together," Oster suggested, urgently, to the technician. A double check on basic procedures was in order.

Within a short time Phillip Brown, evidence in hand, was heading out of the laboratory to obtain a photograph of this abnormal tissue specimen.

Oster was feeling the first faint stirrings of excitement, the itch of intuition. What he was observing was sufficiently strange and unexpected to mean something. Perhaps, warned the cautious scientist in him. Yet it's possible, his optimistic side defended. He had worked long and painstakingly at this program of experiments. Now...suddenly...this could be the light at the end of the tunnel...the breakthrough!

The slide that so puzzled Oster contained a routine specimen tissue. The hospital never informed Oster and his group what type of tissue they had; the material could come from any part of the body. When examined by the naked eye, this particular tissue looked utterly indistinguishable from the myriad other slides that had already been examined. Once stained, however, its unique character was revealed.

Nature's law demanded the presence of the substance called "plasmalogen" in that piece of tissue.

It wasn't there.

Most medical observations are based on what *is* present. What isn't there can often be as important as what is.

The individual cells of the tissues Oster had examined that night were each supposed to contain plasmalogen within the cellular membrane. This particular sample, which Oster later found out to be heart muscle, didn't have a trace of it. Therefore, the sample was not normal, and it was the lack of plasmalogen where it should be which made the sample so significant.

In all his accumulated experiences, Oster had never found anything to match this before. Nor, in fact, had he ever read of such a thing. Later, after a search, he did find reports in the medical literature of similar biochemical changes within atherosclerotic plaques, but none had ever been reported in heart muscle.

It was puzzling because Oster could not think of any reason for the disappearance to have occurred.

Rachel Carson, the author of *Silent Spring*, was equally puzzled when she realized the spring was silent. She finally noticed that the number of robins was diminished.

"Why?" she asked, and exposed chemical pollution.

Carson's work is symbolic of Oster's. Eventually, he was to discover that another type of chemical pollution was responsible for the lack of plasmalogen in cardiovascular tissue.

Oster had many sleepless nights following that perplexing discovery. He kept trying to fit the various discrete pieces of his medical and biochemical evidence together. The answer didn't come but he was, nonetheless, exhilarated.

"I was convinced that somehow, this was the long-awaited breakthrough," he recalled years later, when discussing that momentous occasion in 1964.

A Hypothesis is Created

Slowly, carefully, Oster pieced together the information about the discovery. The history behind that particular piece of heart tissue was important. The organs the trio worked on were supplied from routine hospital autopsies. Oster did not have any prior information about the cause of death of the person from whom the tissue sample had been taken. Now, Oster was impelled to find out as much as possible about the medical history of the person whose tissue it had been.

In the dispassionate language of the report he

eventually published in the *American Journal of Cardiology*, this is the essence of what he unearthed:

> A 51-year old white man was brought to Park City Hospital by car and walked into the Emergency room. He stated that approximately 15 minutes before admission, while at work, he had suddenly experienced severe chest pain which did not radiate in any direction. The patient had not been seriously ill prior to this admission.... The patient was pronounced dead about 40 minutes after admission and 55 minutes after the onset of symptoms. Autopsy was performed approximately one hour after death.... In this one case of myocardial infarction resulting in death within one hour of the onset of symptoms, the plasmalogens disappeared from the focal area of the myocardium, [the muscular tissue of the heart].

Even as he wrote the report, Oster did not understand where it was leading, but he raised the following hypothesis in the discussion and summary of the paper:

> In this case, early disappearance of plasmalogens suggests the possibility that in the early phases of myocardial infarction, perhaps before the occurrence of actual irreversible muscle cell necrosis, an enzyme was liberated. This enzyme then split the plasmalogens, and the resulting plasmal aldehydes diffused into the surrounding tissue and were rapidly oxidized.... The enzyme may have properties similar to those of lecithinase A [now called phospholipase A] to which it might also be related chemically. If this were the case, the possibility exists that the intense pain associated with myocardial infarction may be a manifestation of enzymatic action on the phospholipid-rich myelin sheath of sensory nerve endings in the heart.

More simply put, phospholipase, an enzyme, is dormant within the heart muscle cell. If phospholipase is activated within the confines of a cell, the enzyme immediately attacks the phospholipids within a cell, including those in the cell membrane.

At this point in time, Oster was not sure what factor, or factors, could activate the enzyme. However, the possibility existed that such factors caused plasmalogen in the phospholipid component to seep out of the cell membrane, in somewhat the same way that mortar might flake from a brick wall over a period of time. Researchers use the term "leaky" to describe the state of the damaged membrane. A cell with a leaky membrane has a very short survival time.

A Possible Cause of Angina

The medical community has no proven, biochemically viable explanation for the cause of angina pectoris, or the chest pain associated with heart disease. However, the theory Oster presented in his published study of January 1966 offers a reasonable explanation for at least one cause of angina, namely, a phospholipase attack on the phospholipid component of nerve endings within the heart.

The 1966 paper is, quite literally, the Magna Carta of Oster's work. The information in this first published report by Oster on his developing theory of the origins of a dietary causes of atherosclerosis would, eventually, be clarified and polished by its author. That would take quite a few more years and a great deal more research. Thus, this report was the first attempt at explaining the mysterious disappearance of plasmalogen during a heart attack. It became the foundation of his research.

The tissue that so intrigued Oster by its lack of plasmalogen was put through one of the standard procedures for examining autopsy tissue, one that is performed daily in hospital histology labs throughout the world.

It had first been stained for the purpose of establishing the presence of plasmalogen. However, it was possible that the mysterious disappearance of plasmalogen might have been caused by cellular decomposition prior to autopsy.

On the evening of the discovery the researchers had to resolve a basic yet important question. What was the actual state of the tissue they had examined? If the tissue cells were already dead, or in medical terms, necrotic, upon analysis, then the absence of plasmalogen would be expected. When cells die, the biochemicals in cells go through changes causing the cellular architecture to break down. This makes it very difficult, if not impossible, to distinguish the various cellular components.

Clearly, then, the time sequence was an important factor in the discovery of the disappearance of plasmalogen. Several details had to be checked. Research must always establish, by a careful routine, the precise sequence of the changes being exaimined.

Oster's team had to establish the absence of cell necrosis in the autopsy tissue that fateful evening in November. They took a second tissue block from the same area the first sample had been taken. This time they fixed it in formaldehyde, thus preserving the tissue. Then the sample was sent to the histology-pathology lab for routine staining with hematoxylin and eosin. Oster would not have an answer for forty-eight hours, the time it would take the technicians to complete the staining procedure.

On the night of what later would prove to be a

momentous discovery, Oster left the laboratory slowly, completely preoccupied with the mystery. Usually, his drive home took fifteen minutes. On this particular night, it seemed like seconds, for Oster was methodically reviewing in his mind every single detail of the research work.

He sat in his study, absorbed in his thoughts. In bed, he lay with his eyes shut as he carefully considered what he had to do. It was a sleepless night for Oster.

He *knew* the tissue was different.

He had to find out *why* the tissue was different.

He had to find out *what* the difference meant.

Unmasking The Culprit

Fatigue was kept at bay by Oster's preoccupation with the significance of the previous evening's observations. However, he wasn't overexcited. Years of experience in research had conditioned him to remain detached from his projects. He had to remain cool, impartial.

He went through the hectic morning of hospital rounds at his usual breezy pace, despite the previous night's lack of sleep. Behind his cheery answers and his attention to detail, he was conscious of a growing anxiety as he waited to see the report from the histopathology lab.

Only when the report arrived would he know whether the cellular architecture of the autopsy tissue they had been working on was intact. If the stained tissue revealed the presence of intact nuclei, the first structures to disappear after cells die, the mandate would be clear for Oster to continue with his work. He would search for an explanation for the oddity his team had unveiled; he could proceed assured that his research had promise. He would know in forty-eight hours.

As Oster talked to each patient, he was pain-

fully conscious of the terrible effects of atherosclerosis. Patient after patient on his round displayed the life-debilitating symptoms of the disease. He could identify with the discomfort of his
patients, and he knew very well the course the disease usually took. Would he find a way of preventing or reversing this disease before it struck him
down, too, he wondered?

The Scene of the Crime

The battlefield for atherosclerosis is the arteries.

The circulatory system has blood vessels of
varying diameters. The largest are the arteries, the
smallest are the capillaries. The closed system of
vessels is a continuous network connected to the
heart, which drives the whole system.

By the time a child has grown to maturity, the
circulatory system has 60,000 miles of blood vessels, which, if placed end to end, would stretch two
and one half times around the world or a quarter of
the distance from the earth to the moon.

Although arteries and veins are interdependent
and equally important, the two are structurally and
functionally quite different. The arteries are the
muscular vessels that force, through successive
wave-like contractions, oxygen-rich blood from
the lung via the heart to the various body tissues.
Veins return blood from the periphery of the body
back to the heart. Since veins do not possess a
muscular layer, blood is forced through them by
the pressure gradient created by the movement of
the rib cage when a person inhales and exhales air
and by the contractions of skeletal muscles in the
immediate vicinity of veins. One-way valves in
veins keep venous blood moving in one direction.
Diseases which affect veins are nonatherosclerotic.

Veins are susceptible to blood clots, but they are not prone to the disease processes affecting arteries, unless veins are used as new channels for bypass operations.

Blood leaves the heart through the one inch thick aorta, the main artery, which branches off to the smaller arteries. Arterioles connect the arteries to the narrow capillaries which are as slender as the finest silk threads, only 0.02 inches wide. The small diameter of capillaries forces individual red blood cells to fold over on themselves in order to pass through.

If they are free of disease, arteries are smooth and flexible, in striking contrast to the thicker, more rigid arteries afflicted with arteriosclerosis.

Each artery consists of three primary layers, as illustrated in Figure 1.

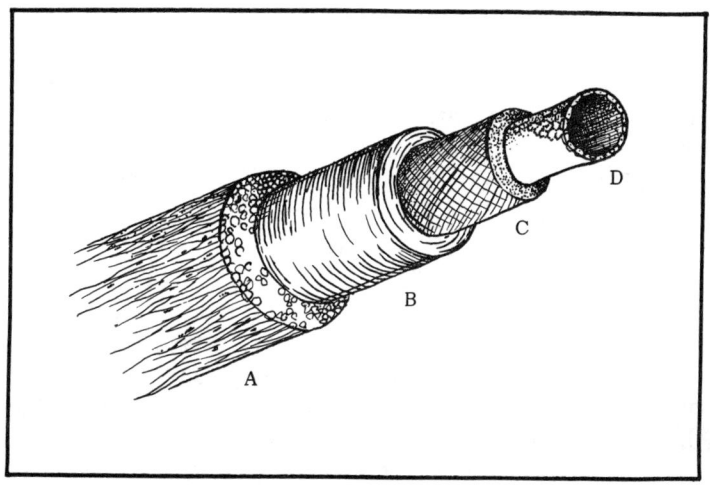

Figure 1. Artery Cross Section
A The outer layer is called the adventitia.
B The middle layer is the media.
C The inner layer is the intima.
D The intima has a lining, the endothelium.

1. The *adventitia* is a loosely packed mix of cells, fibrous protein, and other molecules. It is separated from the next layer, the media, by a grid of elastic fibers, the external elastic lamina.

2. The *media* is a grouping of smooth muscle cells. These contract the artery and counter the stretching produced by any increases in local blood pressure.

3. The *intima* is the innermost grouping of cells in the wall of the artery. Normally, only the intima is in direct contact with blood cells coursing through a vessel.

4. The *endothelium* is a one-cell-thick layer of flattened cells, which lines the intima. It is so thin that its component cells do not pile up but lie next to each other, edges touching.

Atherosclerosis is an odd looking, monstrous word. In Greek, *athere* means porridge or gruel; *sclerosis* means hardening, terms which attempt to describe the consistency of the atherosclerotic plaque which builds in the intima.

Atherosclerosis causes heart attacks and strokes. It contributes to diminished hearing and eyesight. It leads to senility. It cripples and kills. Atherosclerosis is a slow and silent assassin.

Although the terms arteriosclerosis and atherosclerosis are often used interchangeably, a subtle distinction may be drawn between the two diseases. Arteriosclerosis is the abnormal thickening and calcification of the artery wall, which results in a loss of elasticity. Atherosclerosis is the same condition, with the additional accumulation of fatty material in the artery wall.

The term "atherosclerosis" is generally credited to Dr. Felix Marchand in 1904. However, "arteriosclerosis" is believed to have first been coined by a pathologist from Strasbourg, Professor J. E. Lobstein, who introduced the word to the medical profession in the 1930s.

Whether a physician describes the condition as arteriosclerosis or atherosclerosis, how do problems of the cardiovascular system begin?

Any damage to the endothelium can initiate arterial disease. When some element carried by the blood damages and penetrates the artery lining, the smooth muscle cells of the media proliferate in a disorganized fashion much like cancer cells multiplying within a tumor.

In the sad sequence of biochemical events characterizing this leading killer, continuous injury to the artery lining leads progressively to larger lesions and to plaque development within the artery wall between the endothelium and the media layers. Subsequently, plaques may become continuous beneath the endothelial lining. Accumulation of fatty material may take place within plaques. These plaques are then referred to as atheromas. With time, the cells in the interior of an atheroma die off, leaving dead tissue.

Once the lumen of the arteries is narrowed by atheromas, the scene is ripe for disaster. If the passage through which blood flows in an artery is blocked by the "gruel" of atherosclerosis, blood flow is drastically impeded and the heart must work harder to pump the blood through. Sometimes, atheromas become so large that they cause almost total blockage of the flow of blood. At such sites the endothelial lining may tear and blood clots may form. If part of the atheroma is dislodged it travels through the arterial system and lodges in the smaller arteries, a condition known as an embolism. If it is the coronary arteries that are thus affected, the heart may go into spasms and shudder to a stop.

However, in more than half of all cases, death from a heart attack is not swift but is preceded by a host of life-debilitating symptoms. Before the ultimate breakdown, the reduced delivery of blood to organs and tissues produces a host of maladies depending on the tissues affected. They range from diminished eyesight and hearing to kidney failure, from angina chest pain to arterial ulcers of the extremities, from irregularities of the heartbeat to poor leg circulation – all warnings that usually have one cause: diseased arteries.

Atherosclerosis, then, begins with an injury to the endothelium. Oster knew this. So did his colleagues and the rest of the cardiologists in the medical community. But he alone now was very close to discovering and proving the identity of one of the initial damaging agents.

Atherogenesis – Another Perspective On How The Disease Starts

Often discoveries and medical breakthroughs are made when the challenge confronting the scientist is viewed from a fresh angle, from a perspective which may be different and, quite often, not understood and, therefore, not accepted by the uninitiated or untrained mind.

As he sat in the Park City Hospital cafeteria during a short lunch break, Oster's thoughts took him away from the hospital rounds he had just completed. If atherosclerosis starts with an injury to the artery wall, then the disease must be a reaction to injury.

In his mind, Oster attempted to piece together an analogy. A few grains of sand or pebbles in a shoe become out-of-place elements that can precipitate an injury when the shoe is worn. The skin on the foot will redden; it may become raw and very painful. Later in the natural healing process, a scab forms. One can see and feel the sequence of events following an external injury. When a similar reaction occurs in the inner lining of an artery, the lack of nerve endings prevents pain from being registered in the brain.

Yet the body still reacts to the injury. It initiates a repair process.

It made sense to Oster that the onset of atherosclerosis is the body's attempt, over a period of time, to heal its injured arteries. What complicates the healing mechanism, he hypothesized, must be the pebble, which is not removed.

Oster further reasoned that injury to the heart muscle may also occur. Again, the body tries to heal such damage, with the result that internal scar tissue is formed, much like the external scar tissue on someone who has been cut with a knife in an accident.

No matter what causes the injury, the reaction will follow a similar sequence.

Two days after the fateful evening in 1964, Oster was working at his office desk reviewing the accumulated knowledge of cardiology. He opened a textbook, seeking clues about what factor, or factors, may initiate the injury to the artery wall. He read, for perhaps the hundredth time, what had been drilled into him since his first day as a cardiologist.

Injury to the arteries results in the following:

Stage One

Lesions are the first stage in the development of atherosclerosis. An accumulation of fatty streaks, gelatinous lumps and very small blood clots, lesions may occur within all the arteries of the body, including those which nourish the heart, the coronary arteries.

Stages Two and Three

Plaques, which represent the next stage, are formed by an influx of cholesterol esters, fibrin, platelets, and calcium — the amounts will vary. In the final stage, as plaques grow, ulceration, calcification, hemorrhages, and blood clots may develop.

Oster made careful note of the absence of cholesterol in the first stage of atherosclerosis, despite the popular claims of those assuring the public that cholesterol in food initiates atherosclerosis. The hearse before the horse, he mused.

A knock at the door brought Oster out of his chair. Nurse O'Neill had not yet come in that morning. Was it she or the results from pathology? Phillip Brown was at the door. He waved a large manila envelope.

"Confirmed," he exclaimed with restrained excitement. "The pathology report confirms the tissue was not necrotic even though it lacked plasmalogen."

Oster glanced out the window at the early morning sunlight. They had definitely stumbled on the brink of a discovery. Time, and more work, would show its importance. Now he would dig as deep as needed to understand the mystery.

Revelations of an Important Kind

The cornerstone of Oster's theory had been laid with that historical autopsy study in 1964. He had been alert enough, and informed enough, to recognize that the baffling lack of plasmalogen from the heart muscle was significant.

In his mind, Oster reviewed over and over again the data and information which he had accumulated over the years in the course of his study of chemistry, clinical pharmacology, and laboratory research.

Initially, Oster and his team were not told the anatomical site of the autopsy tissue. When Oster decided to check into the background of the autopsy material, he found that it came from a 51-year-old man who had died, with hideous speed, of a heart attack.

Before the fatal attack, however, the victim had not displayed any of the symptoms normally associated with heart and circulatory disease. Another intriguing fact was that the pathology study of the heart muscle did not show the scarring usually associated with atherosclerosis, even though the electrocardiogram presented changes characteristic of a myocardial infarction.

The subsequent study – one which supported, but was curiously different from, the 1964 work – involved an examination of more autopsy tissue. This time, it involved a youngster who was killed while speeding on his motorbike. He overshot a curve on a bridge, hitting and vaulting a guard rail, and precipitating himself into the watery depths of Long Island Sound.

In this, the second study, the tissues analyzed were from an apparently healthy 22-year-old male whose death was accidental. The intriguing aspect of this study was the absence of plasmalogen from the inner lining of the aorta, even though the young man did not die from a heart attack. This was most startling. Figure 2. shows the aorta of this drowning victim with the earliest changes that take place in the initial phases of atherosclerosis.

The bottom left light gray area is the interior cavity of the aorta. Plasmalogen has disappeared from behind the intact intima. The darkish material infiltrating the area where plasmalogen has dis-

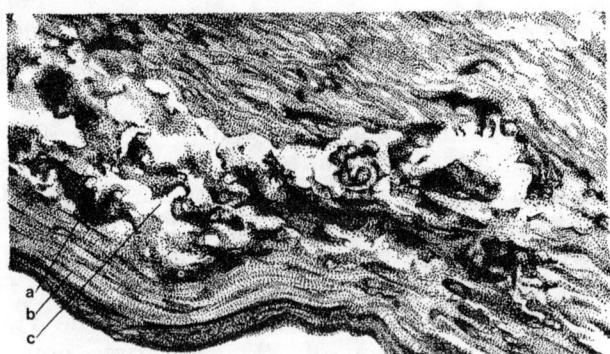

Figure 2. Aorta of 22-Year-Old Apparently Healthy Drowning Victim. Lesion behind intact intima. Cross section 480X. (a) cholesterol, neutral fat, and fibrous tissue. (b) intact intima; inner artery wall. (c) depleted plasmalogen. Photo-Oster.

appeared most likely consists of cholesterol esterified with monounsaturated acid. Even though he was an apparently healthy 22-year-old who had never shown any clinical signs of atherosclerosis, the pronounced changes in his artery were characteristic of the initial phases of atherosclerosis.

Once the second study was completed, Oster had two sets of facts. Each had been discovered independently of the other. Yet somehow, Oster believed, each was inextricably linked. He was determined to find the connection.

Questions in Search of Solutions

The puzzling question of what caused the mysterious disappearance of plasmalogen perplexed the research team. It was a seemingly bizarre phenomenon that had repeated itself in two isolated instances. It might have been involved in the death of an apparently healthy person.

By drawing on his store of specialized information, Oster began to outline the shape of a possible culprit. The enzyme xanthine oxidase, known as XO for short, came under suspicion, for it is a substance found in virtually every animal, including humans.

The available facts were scattered and pitifully few.

"This one piece of evidence," Oster would eventually recall, "the absence of plasmalogen in the heart attack victim and later in the young drowning victim, seemed to be a significant clue. Yet it was a clue floating alone, disconnected from any helpful information.

"If it hadn't been for the fortunate coincidence of my work at Columbia University almost three decades earlier, I might never have made the connection.

"You see, the enzyme called xanthine oxidase can oxidize, or change, plasmalogen to a different substance. If this had happened in the tissue we were examining, it would have seemed as if the plasmalogen had disappeared because it didn't show the normal result when we stained it with fuchsin sulfurous acid, the Feulgen stain.

"Perhaps, I asked myself, the xanthine oxidase which our own body produces is reponsible for plasmalogen's disappearance? After all, the liver produces xanthine oxidase.

"At first it seemed a logical explanation. But, two fallacies in this argument soon became evident. XO is one of the many enzymes manufactured by the body; it is endogenous. Why would an endogenous enzyme attack another part of a person? Also, under normal circumstances one should never find XO in heart or aorta tissue because XO and plasmalogen are usually not found together in the same tissue. Chemically, the two are as incompatible as a cat and a canary. I began to have doubts that it could be the body's own XO that was responsible for plasmalogen depletion. I puzzled for some time over the possible connection.

"One day it dawned on me how to resolve this fundamental question. I realized the offending XO might originate from outside the body. That suggested diet. I knew that much of the food we eat, whether from plants or animals, also contains xanthine oxidase.

"My investigation now had two well-defined targets. I first had to prove whether XO was a culprit. If it was, I had to establish its source."

In order to avoid wasting precious time and money, researchers first thoroughly scan all available literature on the subject under investigation when starting a project. Oster's literature search revealed that the absence of XO in normal human cardiac tissues had been reported by E. J. Morgan as far back as 1926. Oster then remembered he had actually utilized this relatively obscure information in his work with Dr. Michael Mulinos at Columbia University nearly thirty years ago. Oster pulled the paper, which had been published in 1944, out of his files.

"What did we use to show how plasmalogen could be changed?" he asked himself as he skimmed over his original paper.

"Aha, here it is. As I thought. It was XO!"

In this paper, Oster and Mulinos explained that the presence of XO in certain parts of the body, most notably in the liver and in the mucous membrane of the small intestine, was directly responsible for the natural absence of plasmalogen from the cell membrane at these sites.

He recalled how he had started the study at

Columbia by obtaining a sample of rare, purified XO from the laboratory of the famous biochemist, D. E. Green, and how cautiously he worked with it. In those days, refining XO was exceedingly costly, and research dollars were scarce in this area.

As Oster put aside his original research paper, he decided to repeat some of his earlier findings. He spent several weeks examining the chemical effects of XO on living tissue cultures in the lab (in vitro) to confirm the chemical reaction between XO and plasmalogen which he had witnessed twenty-six years earlier with Mulinos.

But this was not enough. He now had to be able to identify the presence of XO in living tissues. This was not an area where Oster had technical expertise. He was at a roadblock, but he was not about to turn back. He decided his next study must, somehow, establish XO's presence at the scene of the crime.

A Meeting of Minds

Good fortune then brought Oster and Dr. Donald Ross together. It was a serendipitous encounter.

"My first meeting with Donald Ross was in 1969, just after Thanksgiving, at a directors' meeting of our local Heart Association.

"I'm almost certain I remember our first conversation verbatim," Oster added as he recalled that initial meeting with Donald Ross.

"When we were introduced, I thought to myself that Ross looked the part of the college professor. The quintessential teacher. Casual tweed jacket. Pipe. Once you start talking to him, you find his relaxed manner cloaks a razor-keen mind. Quite energetic. He finds time to teach several sections of biology a semester, and handle administrative work, as well as to conduct an active research program.

"The president of the Greater Bridgeport Heart Association made the introduction," Oster recalled.

"Doctor Oster, this is Doctor Ross, Chairman of the Department of Biology at Fairfield University, our latest Board Member," the president said.

"Doctor Oster, one of our founding directors, who has been a member since 1949," he continued. "Welcome."

Oster shook hands with Ross.

For a few moments the three discussed the meeting, then the president moved away.

Oster and Ross fell into casual conversation.

"How long have you been at Fairfield University?"

"Since 1950. Almost twenty years now."

Oster listened as Ross described the courses he taught.

"I'm a Health Sciences Advisor, so I act more or less as a consultant, a support system, for various disciplines. I teach comparative anatomy, biophysics, cell physiology, and biochemistry."

Oster's interest heightened at the mention of the other's specialities. He started to discuss his work. "I've been concentrating my research, what time I have for it, in one particular area since 1964," he said. "As a cardiologist, I'm interested in identifying a dietary cause of atherosclerosis. All this talk of cholesterol being the culprit in atherosclerotic health problems is on the wrong track, as far as I'm concerned."

Ross nodded in agreement. "All the drugs to lower serum cholesterol haven't worked. The single risk factor theory is bankrupt."

Delighted with the informed response, Oster took the initiative.

"I had an article in *Cardiology Digest*, 'Treatment of Angina Pectoris According to a New Theory of Its Origin'."

When Oster sensed Ross had not seen the article he promised to send him a reprint.

"I need to know more about the enzyme xanthine oxidase, XO. I've searched the literature and there doesn't seem to be much more than I've already unearthed."

In the pause that followed, the two men looked at each other thoughtfully. Ross finished packing his pipe and was about to speak when Oster asked a question.

"Actually, it's quite a coincidence meeting you today, because I did turn up a reference to some work done by someone at your place, Fairfield University. Perhaps you can help me track him down."

"You have," came the reply.

"Excuse me?"

"Tracked me down. My doctoral dissertation was on xanthine oxidase in Japanese beetles."

Oster was astounded. He did not hesitate. His next words were aimed at the most important step in his research.

"But can you measure XO in cardiovascular tissues?" he queried Ross.

"Sure. You can measure it in anything!"

The hunt was on. Ross not only had an unusual fund of knowledge on XO, but he could resist neither the scientific challenge nor the intellectual stimulation. The collaboration between Doctors Oster and Ross began.

As Lawrence K. Altman, M.D., once noted in the *New York Times*:

> Stories of medical advances often are told as if logic had dictated every step, as if the researchers had known from the beginning what they were looking for and exactly how to find it.

Clearly some developments do reflect logical deductions from planned research. But the development process also involves such nonscientific factors as perseverance and luck. Researchers have discovered new therapies, for example, by: drawing new conclusions from accidental findings; paying attention to the observations of patients; turning unwanted side effects into something of value, and finding new uses for old drugs.

Ross soon devised a study to test Oster's hypothesis that XO might be present in the injured portion of arterial tissue. In the study he decided to compare normal appearing aorta tissue sections with sections which had obvious fatty degeneration (atherosclerotic plaques) in five deceased males. It was decided that the technician handling the actual tissue analysis would not be informed whether tissue samples came from healthy or diseased arteries. This was done to eliminate the technician's prejudice, which could have been a source of error.

The tissue samples were meticulously prepared. They were then all analyzed. Any possible XO activity in the samples was measured by the fluorometer, one of the sensitive instruments sometimes used for this type of work. Eventually, after the lengthy and complex procedures were complete, the critical moment arrived.

Anxiously, Oster and Ross waited and watched. Sure enough, they found that those tissue samples sectioned from diseased areas of arteries not only contained XO but also that the XO that was present was still very much biologically active.

Ross and the premedical student assistant Michael Ptaszynski then performed dozens upon dozens of assays and tests on other artery tissue samples taken from the same five individuals. Their labor was rewarded. The discovery was a scientific first. Until this work at Fairfield University, the scientific world was not aware that XO might be present in diseased arteries and in heart muscle tissue.

Why would anyone even bother to look?

Oster's discovery was, in some ways, reminiscent of the historic search for Pluto. No one had ever "discovered" the existence of the ninth and most distant planet from the sun because no one had ever suspected it was there until an astronomer stumbled upon a clue. Percival Lowell, on the basis of disturbances he observed in the orbit of the planet Neptune, began searching for the planet in 1905. Pluto's presence was confirmed in 1930.

Scientists have been aware for some time that XO and plasmalogen are chemically incompatible. For this reason no one had ever searched for XO in plasmalogen-rich artery tissue. In some ways the finding was a little like discovering an Eskimo settlement in the Sahara. Shockingly out of place.

Shocking or not, the study was a pivotal one. The results were reported in the *Proceedings of the Society For Experimental Biology and Medicine* in 1973. The title is direct: "The Presence of Ectopic Xanthine Oxidase in Atherosclerotic Plaques and Myocardial Tissues" (ectopic means out of place).

Enzymes normally serve many useful functions. One is the digestion of food in the stomach. However, the enzyme XO does untold damage when it is in an alien location such as an artery and heart muscle tissue. XO speeds up, or catalyzes, a specific chemical reaction in which the aldehydes in plasmalogen are oxidized. Probably, there are other mechanisms by which XO can deplete the natural reservoir of plasmalogen in the body, but hard evidence to support this possibility is lacking.

The paper presented by Oster and Ross in 1973 might have raised more questions than it answered. But this is not uncommon in science. Discoveries often unlock a Pandora's box of new questions; eventually, advances are made as answers to the questions are found. In the conclusion of the report, Oster and Ross made a most intriguing suggestion about the possible source of the XO isolated in the autopsy tissues.

Since normal human serum does not contain XO, Oster and Ross proposed two possible sources.

> One source of the enzyme XO may be the liver cells, since patients with acute liver disease show increased serum levels of xanthine oxidase. Also, in patients with chronic liver disease, the serum level of xanthine oxidase is occasionally moderately elevated. Moreover, in uncomplicated...jaundice, the serum xanthine oxidase is, at times, slightly elevated....
>
> Another potential source of the enzyme XO...bovine milk is presently under investigation in this laboratory since it has been shown that milk antibodies are significantly elevated in the blood of male patients with ischemic heart disease. [Where the supply of oxygen is insufficient to a tissue, the problem is called ischemic.]

With the publication of this study in 1973, Oster made it clear to his colleagues that he was no longer a member of the cholesterol and dietary fat fraternity. To a few, it seemed an intelligent choice. To the majority, it was heresy. Those researchers who implicated cholesterol and other risk factors as the cause of atherosclerosis were riding high in the 1970s. It is not surprising that after the Oster-Ross paper was published, critics became more numerous and increasingly vocal. Such critics pointed out that drawing conclusions from an experiment involving tissue samples from only five persons was not reliable.

Oster and Ross did not have the money to pay for similar lab work on a larger scale. That would involve analyzing thousands of autopsy tissue samples. However, their work was accurate scientific research. Any laboratory anywhere in the world could duplicate the test and find the same abnormality, a lack of plasmalogen in atherosclerotic tissues. Even a single abnormality can shed new light on an old problem. The findings of Oster and Ross should be considered as significant, if not more so, than the deductions drawn by epidemiologists from studies involving unrelated population groups.

The Nutrition Council of the American Heart Association soon entered the picture. They suggested that XO in arterial tissue came from the body's supply in the liver.

Oster and Ross did not find it easy to accept the pronouncement of the Nutrition Council for two fundamental reasons.

First the laws of nature are such that man and other living organisms rarely release chemicals which lead to the destruction of their own tissues. If anything, the body has a tendency towards self-preservation, not self-destruction.

Autoimmune disease, in which the body's own white blood cells destroy one's own tissues, is an exception to this rule, but in this disease, white blood cells are responsible for the damage for a very specific reason: white blood cells destroy any tissue in which the surface characteristics become chemically altered (this makes them appear foreign to white blood cells). White blood cells are programmed to seek out and destroy any foreign tissue, such as transformed cancerous cells, a fact that complicates organ transplantation.

Oster and Ross knew of no reason for XO to pass from one part of the body to another location, in this case the arteries, and wreak havoc there. Perhaps in cases of rare liver disease, XO might seep out, but it is highly unlikely to happen in the average healthy individual who does not have a history of liver disease.

Second Oster had accumulated evidence of another, more likely source of the XO.

When Oster originally considered XO as a possible culprit, he had asked himself the leading question: What widely consumed food contains XO in large quantities?

Chicken and calves liver have XO. However, these foods are usually cooked. Cooking destroys XO. Oster's search revealed that cow's milk has high levels of XO. In fact, cow's milk is the most widely consumed food containing XO. For this reason, Oster decided to accumulate evidence to help establish a possible link between XO in cow's milk and the depletion of XO in artery wall tissue. He suspected this might be one of the initial phases of atherosclerosis.

By drinking the milk of the cow, a food intended for unweaned calves, man is, in effect, tampering with nature. Might the XO health hazard be the consequence of this violation? Certain facts suggested otherwise to Oster. After all, milk has been drunk ever since the domestication of the cow, and by many civilizations. The epidemic of atherosclerosis, however, is something very recent. Could some other factor be held accountable? Through an unusual set of circumstances, Oster stumbled upon the answer.

In 1967, the FDA questioned the quality of chloromycetin, one of the antibiotics manufactured by McKesson. In his official capacity as clinical pharmacologist for McKesson Laboratory, Oster went to Washington to appear before the FDA.

The FDA's accusation was puzzling to Oster.

They maintained that McKesson's chloromycetin was ineffective because it wasn't being distributed in the body as effectively as the chloromycetin manufactured by Parke Davis. Yet each company used identical chemical formulations. McKesson was faced with the possibility of recalling half a million dollars worth of the antibiotic. Even worse, if they could not resolve the problem, McKesson would have to stop manufacturing the drug.

It did not take Oster long to pinpoint the source of the problem. The chloromycetin crystals in the two products were of different sizes. The Parke Davis crystals were micronized, or considerably smaller than the McKesson crystals. This is an important difference, for a fine powder is absorbed more efficiently into the body than a coarse one.

Micronization...homogenization.... Oster was absorbed in thought during the flight back to New York's LaGuardia Airport. Could this possibly apply to his work on XO? Could the homogenization of milk somehow be increasing the biological availability of XO for passage into one's circulatory system in the same way the micronization of the Parke Davis drug increased its uptake from the gut? As he walked off the plane, he sensed he had converted adversity into profit for his theory. He would try to tie in the lesson learned in Washington to support his hypothesis that the homogenization of milk may increase the biological availability of XO.

Around the World in Search of Facts

Even before Oster met Ross and suggested that they search for the presence of XO in tissue from arteries, he had confirmed his suspicions that the XO might come from a source outside the body. In Oster's opinion, homogenized milk was the culprit, and he had gathered some facts to support this. The material was actually statistical, and Oster knew he could not rely on it totally, but it did offer some interesting evidence.

He had collected figures from thirteen different countries. His sources were embassies and government bureaus, the World Health Organization, the American National Dairy Council in Chicago, the Department of Agriculture in Washington, and dairy institutes in other countries. He put all the information into a chart that compared two subjects:

1. Death rates from atherosclerotic and degenerative heart disease, per 100,000 people

   with

2. Consumption of milk, butter, and cheese

The statistics gathered showed extremely interesting patterns. Oster was quick to observe that milk consumption correlated with the prevalence of atherosclerosis while the consumption of butter

Table 1. Comparison of death rates per 100,000 population from atherosclerotic and degenerative heart disease with consumption of milk and dairy products

Country	1967 Death Rate	Pounds Per Person Fluid Milk Intake	Pounds Per Person		Relative Standing			Homog- enized	Pre Boiled Frequently
			Butter	Cheese	M	B	C		
1. Finland	244.7	593	35.	7.3	1	1	12	⅓	No
2. United States	211.8	273	4.7	10.6	9	11	7	almost all	No
3. Australia	204.6	304	22.9	7.8	7	2	11	not generally	?
4. Canada	187.4	288	16.2	9.0	8	8	9	partially	No
5. United Kingdom	140.9	350	19.7	11.0	4	4	6	about 7½%	No
6. Netherlands	106.9	337	5.7	19.5	5	10	4	infrequently	?
7. F.R. of Germany	102.3	213	18.7	9.3	11	5	8	partially	?
8. Austria	88.6	327	13.2	8.4	6	9	10	occasionally	?
9. Sweden	74.7	374	16.3	18.3	2	7	5	?	Yes
10. Italy	78.9	137	4.0	19.9	6	12	3	12.5%	Yes
11. Switzerland	75.9	370	16.4	22.1	3	6	2	small quantity	Yes
12. France	41.7	230	19.9	28.8	10	3	1	negligible	Yes
13. Japan	39.1	48	?	?				occasionally	?

Death rates (45–54-year-old men). Source: World Health Statistics Annual, World Health, Aug.–Sept issue. p. 11, 1970.
Consumption of fluid milk and cream, butter, and cheese in selected foreign countries, 1968. Source: W. T. Butz, How Americans Use Their Dairy Foods, National Dairy Council, Chicago, Ill., p. 15, 1970.

and cheese had little to do with the prevalence of the disease. Since Oster had only recently escaped from the confines of the cholesterol and dietary fat school of thought, he was quite intrigued with the results of his survey.

In Japan, where milk is not as widely consumed as in Western countries, the death rate from atherosclerosis and degenerative heart disease is exceptionally low.

France had five times fewer deaths from circulatory disease than did the United States, even though the French per capita intake of butter and cheese was 3.25 times greater.

Finland, which showed the highest consumption of fluid milk in the world, had a correspondingly high death rate and was at the top of the list of the thirteen countries surveyed.

For most scientists, milk is milk. Oster's background in pharmacology and his recent experience in Washington helped him look at milk from a different perspective. He put yet another entry into Table 1. He compared whether milk was homogenized, raw or preboiled in each country.

Countries where most of the milk used is homogenized, such as the United States, consistently displayed the highest death rates from atherosclerosis and degenerative heart disease. It was becoming increasingly obvious to Oster that the homogenization of milk had some significance.

Is Milk a Natural?

By the time milk reaches the family refrigerator, pasteurization and homogenization have altered milk's physical properties so that it only vaguely resembles the natural product. Homogenization and pasteurization are two of the most common processing steps that milk is put through. Depending on the type of processing, milk and dairy products contain varying amounts of potentially damaging XO. Although pasteurization and homogenization are quite different, their meanings are often confused.

Pasteurization

The process of pasteurization is named after the French chemist, Louis Pasteur. The process is utilized to achieve the partial sterilization of liquids, especially milk, wine, and beer, for the purpose of destroying disease-causing organisms, for reducing total bacteria counts, and eliminating enzymes responsible for producing off-flavors.

A June 1982, article in *Consumers Reports*, "Milk, Could It Taste Better?" explains that in limits set by the U.S. Public Health Service, milk fresh from the pasteurizer "should contain no more than 20,000 bacteria and 10 coliform fecal organisms per milliliter." The article claims the allowed numbers are far too high and the journal suggests limits of 2,000 bacteria per milliliter and zero for coliform bacteria.

In the United States and some other countries until the late 1970s, milk was pasteurized by heating it to about 140° Fahrenheit (63° C) for 30 minutes, followed by rapid cooling to below 50° Fahrenheit (10° C). The milk was then stored at this temperature. Most dairies in the United States now use a higher heat with a shorter holding period. Some, not all, of the XO is inactivated by pasteurization, roughly 42 percent.

Although some XO remains in pasteurized, nonhomogenized milk, (where it is found in association with the exterior of the milk fat globule membrane) the chances that the enzyme will be taken up from the gut are decreased, since large fat globules are less likely to pass with XO through the intestinal wall into the circulation.

UHT Pasteurization

In January 1982, the Federal Drug Administration approved a technology that could help change milk processing around the world — if consumers can be persuaded to live with the cooked taste it produces.

Ultra-High Temperature (UHT) processing sterilizes milk and milk products by first using high temperatures and then quickly bringing down the temperature. This effectively destroys bacteria that could cause spoilage. Industry spokesmen claim "the process also preserves more flavor and nutrients than other methods." However, since heat destroys heat-labile vitamins in milk, there is room for argument.

UHT milk is packaged in a five-layer container that is impervious to bacteria. Manufacturers say it safely holds fluid milk on pantry shelves for up to three months without refrigeration.

Today, some of the milk in countries such as Japan, West Germany, France, and Switzerland is ultrapasteurized. This milk is heated to a temperature of 93.3°C, which irreversibly inactivates XO.

Homogenization

Homogenization is the process in which the particle size of a mixture is made uniform throughout. This procedure involves reducing the size of the fat particles in the cream portion of milk and dispersing them evenly throughout the rest of the milk by forcing milk at high speeds through a fine filter at the enormous pressure of 4,500 pounds per square inch.

The practice of homogenizing milk became widespread in the U.S. in the 1930s for the purpose of slightly extending the shelflife of the product.

This increased two things: cost to the consumer and profit for stores and for milk manufacturers. When milk has not been homogenized, the globules of fat vary in size and are relatively large, which allows them to separate and rise to the top of milk.

Most people still remember how before homogenization became widespread, cream in milk used to rise to the top of the bottle. Today, one can still observe the same phenomenon in raw milk, which is occasionally available from small farms, dairies, and health food stores. Naturally, producers of raw milk must comply with the same stringent regulations that govern other milk producers. Many of these small producers of raw milk have superior establishments that not only comply with but exceed state requirements.

Today, in the 1980s, the bulk of milk distributed in westernized countries, including the United States, is both pasteurized and homogenized.

Oster's research shows that homogenization causes the specific change in particle size which allows XO to pass through the intestinal wall into the circulatory system. After homogenization the fat globules are reduced to one-third their original size, while their surface area more than triples. Fat remains evenly dispersed in milk because of the altered surface characteristics of fat globules.

XO, which is found along the exterior of the milk fat globule membrane before homogenization, is encapsulated during the homogenization process by the new lipoprotein membrane, an artifact of the homogenization process. This membrane consists of fats, phospholipids, and casein and is more resistant to digestion than the original milk fat globule membrane. It protects XO within the newly created vehicle against the influence of some of the digestive enzymes and allows some XO to pass intact from the gut into the circulatory system.

circulatory system.

Stomach acid, which is strong enough to destroy XO, is neutralized by the strong buffering properties of milk. One glass of milk is sufficient to buffer stomach acid, so that much of the XO is not inactivated.

Oster reported in 1978 that the fat droplets called liposomes could cross the intestinal barrier undigested. Ultimately, some of these droplets enter the circulating blood, where their lipoprotein membranes appear to be digested by the enzyme lipoprotein lipase, which is located in capillary linings. Thus, the previously protected XO is made biologically available which means XO can be absorbed by the body.

The evidence Oster gathered in his original survey of thirteen nations provided interesting support of his theory that homogenized cow's milk might be the culprit in the atherosclerotic process. Soon additional evidence fell into place and rewarded Oster's persistence.

Full Circle

After the Ross team at Fairfield University discovered XO in atherosclerotic plaques and in artery tissue which was devoid of plasmalogen, several challenging questions remained.

First, conclusive proof had to be found that XO was not endogenous, that it was not seeping out of the liver into the circulatory system, as some critics maintained. Second, it was necessary to establish that XO in the arteries was from cow's milk. Oster and Ross needed more reliable proof than epidemiology.

In order to resolve these two important questions, Oster and his team used a clever and highly reliable method for determining the source of the XO. Antibodies in the bloodstream serve as a line of defense against the chemicals released by viruses and bacteria. Each antibody is highly specific and is formed in response to a particular foreign substance. Because of the specificity of antibodies, it is possible to identify, with considerable accuracy, which foreign substance has been present, and in what quantity, in the blood. The team set about analyzing the blood of volunteers for the presence of an antibody against XO from cow's milk.

"Immune Response to Bovine Xanthine Oxidase in Atherosclerotic Patients," the double blind study published in *American Laboratory* in 1974, was a big step towards substantiating Oster's theory.

In this study, Oster's nurse Barbara O'Neill recruited 75 patients at random from Oster's internal medicine/cardiology practice. She included those patients with clinical signs of atherosclerosis as well as those with no such signs. Each patient's serum would be tested for antibody response to bovine milk xanthine oxidase (BMXO) — but the researchers conducting the study, including Oster, his son, and Ross, would be "blind" on background information about the patients. All they would know is that they had 75 tubes of human sera; only Nurse O'Neill would know which results came from which patients. This would assure the integrity of the study. Only after the analysis of the blood samples would patients be matched with their respective blood samples.

Defining the Ground Rules

Nurse O'Neill recalls how Oster had methodically explained the procedure for the study. "Only one person, you in this case, will have any knowledge of which result matches which patient in this double blind experiment."

"It's the only way I can be certain the results

won't be subject to my personal bias. Because this test is so vital to my research, I obviously have a particular interest in the results turning out a certain way. If I were to choose the participants and if I then collected the results, I might – consciously or unconsciously – influence the results."

She had nodded in understanding.

"It's essential that neither I nor Doctor Ross, who's supervising the lab work, nor the patients will have any information about which patients provided which blood samples."

"Your son, Jeff, is working in the lab with Doctor Ross, but I suppose he won't know any more than you which results belong to which patient?" she had asked.

"Correct," Oster added as he turned and sat down at his desk.

"Anyone involved with the test will be 'blind' on background information," he continued. "Only we and the technicians will know that we have seventy-five tubes of human sera. Each blood sample will be tested for its level of antibody against XO, the results analyzed and then recorded. But let's talk about setting up the experiment. You have the responsibility of recruiting patients, at random. In other words, enlist them from the group of people who come in to see me, for whatever reason," Oster explained.

"Even if they don't have health problems caused by atherosclerosis?" she had queried.

"Not quite."

She had listened attentively as the physician explained the ground rules for the study.

"We have to divide patients into two groups. One group should consist of those who have known signs of atherosclerosis; anything from chest pain to heart attacks. In the other group we will include people who do not have any symptoms of atherosclerosis."

Oster's practice covers internal medicine, his subspecialty is cardiology. People come to his office for a variety of reasons ranging from routine physicals or insurance checkups to serious heart or circulatory problems. The nurse knew she would have no difficulty enlisting a broad range of individuals for the study.

"One last question, doctor. Is it all right to explain to the patients what we're trying to do?"

"Absolutely."

"Fine. I'll tell anyone who is curious that we're checking their antibody response to BMXO, xanthine oxidase in homogenized cow's milk."

"Then they definitely won't know what we're up to," Oster chuckled. "Keep it simple and just tell them we're investigating a method for finding out whether somebody might be a candidate for atherosclerosis."

Oster had then added, "Once we've analyzed the patients' blood for XO, we can breach the anonymity of the blood samples and match them to the proper patients."

Within the next few weeks, the nurse recruited 75 people for the study. Some had been Oster's patients for years. Others were newcomers.

Part of the value and the beauty of the 1974 double blind study was the way it brought Oster's work full cycle by answering several of the key questions that had been unanswered up to this point. Not only did it prove the existence of human XO antibodies from cow's milk, but it also demonstrated a possible connection between the quantity, or titer, of XO antibodies and the extent to which a person was afflicted with atherosclerosis triggered by BMXO.

The graph that follows shows that most patients with no clinical signs of atherosclerosis had a relatively weak antibody reaction to BMXO (shown by the dotted line, from left to right). On a scale of 0 − 5, the reading of 2 is quite low; it suggests that the circulatory systems of these patients have had very little exposure to BMXO.

Patients with proven atherosclerosis showed strong antibody reactions to BMXO (shown by the solid line). The solid line peaks farther to the right than does the dotted line, at a reading of 4 on the scale of 0 − 5. This high agglutination reaction reading indicates that the circulatory systems of these patients have had extensive exposure to BMXO.

The shaded, gray area on the chart has invaluable clinical significance. People whose antibody reactions fall into the gray area on the chart have no symptoms of atherosclerosis yet their XO antibody levels show they have the disease somewhere in their systems on a subclinical level.

Figure 3. Immunoassay of serum xanthine oxidase.

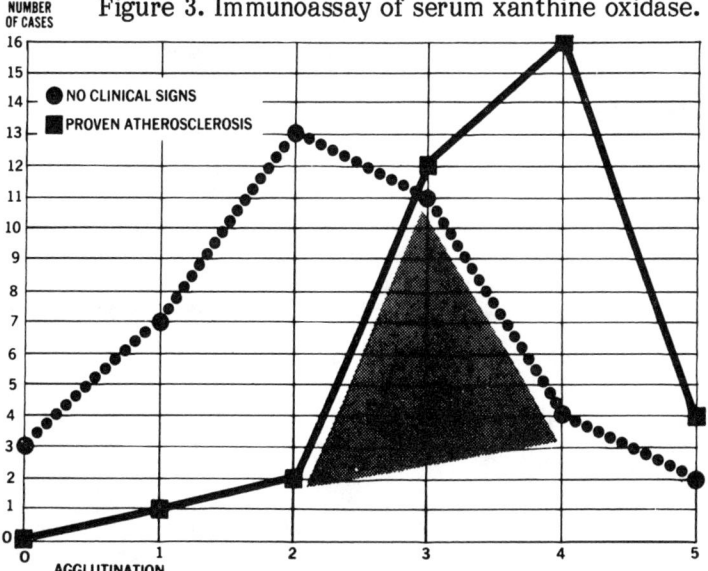

Traditional physicals and checkups cannot detect atherosclerosis until the disease is advanced. The XO antibody test, a powerful screening and diagnostic tool, answers the most common question: "How can I establish what condition of my arteries? Do I have the disease?" The XO antibody test is inexpensive, quick, and not fraught with often serious complications, as are some other diagnostic methods.

In summary, the antibody study reinforced ev-

Table 2

Antibody response to milk proteins and bovine xanthine oxidase in blood serum of patients with no clinical manifestations of atherosclerosis

No.	Sex	Age	Antibody titer milk protein	Antibody titer xanthine oxidase	Diagnosis	Remarks
1	M	71	2	3	Rheum. H. D.ª	Atrial fibrillation
2	M	59	3	3	Neuritis	
3	F	21	2	4		1 qt. of milk daily
4	F	60	0	1	Diab. mell.ᵇ	Hypertension
5	M	72	1	1		
6	F	76	1	1.5	Diab. mell.	Hypertension
7	F	24	1	1		Goat's milk
8	M	28	0	1		Raw cow's milk
9	F	24	1.5	2		
10	M	29	0	0		
11	M	59	1	2	Rheum. H. D.	
12	M	40	2	2		
13	M	71	2	2	Polycythemia	Venous thrombosis
14	M	63	2	2.5	Rheum. H. D.	Aortic stenosis
15	F	57	1	1	Neurosis	
16	M	63	3	2	Hypertension	
17	M	67	3	2	Hypertension	
18	M	48	3.5	5		
19	M	45	3	4	Hypertension	
20	M	58	2	3	Hypertension	
21	F	67	3	2	Rheum. H. D.	Atrial fibrillation
22	M	29	3	1		Boiled buffalo milk
23	F	22	3.5	5	Gastroenteritis	Boiled buffalo milk
24	F	57	1	0		
25	F	47	3	5		
26	M	47	3	3.5		
27	M	68	2	3		
28	M	57	1	0		Possible adrenal tumor. Boiled milk
29	M	38	1	2.5		
30	F	43	2	2		
31	M	68	2	1	Hypertension	
32	F	68	2	3		
33	F	67	2	2		
34	F	46	3	3		
35	F	66	3	2	Diab. mell.	
36	M	70	3	2	Diab. mell.	Hypertension
37	F	62	3	3		
38	F	74	2	3	Arthritis	
39	F	44	3	3		
40	M	29	2	2		
41	F	47	3	5	Peptic ulcer	Gastrectomy

ªRheum. H. D. = rheumatic heart disease.   ᵇDiab. mell. = diabetes mellitus.

ery aspect of Oster's theory while establishing the following points:

- XO from cow's milk (BMXO) may be absorbed and may enter the cardiovascular system.
- Differences in BMXO antibody levels exist from person to person.
- People with clinical signs of atherosclerosis have greater quantities of BMXO antibodies.
- BMXO antibodies are found in greater quanti-

Table 3

Antibody response to milk proteins and bovine xanthine oxidase in blood serum of patients with atherosclerotic diseases

No.	Sex	Age	Antibody response to milk protein	xanthine oxidase	Diagnosis	Remarks
1	M	63	3	3	M. I.[a]	
2	M	39	3	4	M. I.	Angina pectoris. Coronary bypass
3	M	72	2	3.5	M. I.	
4	M	34	4	4	M. I.	
5	M	68	2.5	3.5	M. I.	
6	M	39	2.5	3	M. I.	
7	M	62	2	3.5	Angina pectoris	Coronary arteriography
8	F	60	3	3	M. I.	
9	M	60	2	4	M. I.	Angina pectoris. Psoriasis
10	M	50	2	4	M. I.	
11	M	61	2	3.5	M. I.	Diab. mell.
12	M	64	2	3	M. I.	Diab. mell.
13	M	59	1	3.5	Arrhythmia	
14	F	70	2	4	Claudication	
15	M	69	2	3	C. V. A.[b]	
16	M	60	2.5	4	M. I.	
17	M	62	2.5	4	M. I.	Diab. mell.
18	M	45	2	4	M. I.	
19	M	55	3	3	M. I.	Angina pectoris
20	F	72	2	3	Diab. mell.	Hypertension
21	F	37	2.5	3.5	Renal arter.[d]	Malignant hypertension. Gastrectomy
22	M	69	3	3.5	M. I.	Emphysema
23	M	71	2	2	Claudication	Diab. mell.
24	F	75	3	3	Brain ischemia	Hypertension. Pulmonary embolism
25	F	62	3.5	3	Brain ischemia	
26	F	55	3	1	M. I.	
27	M	63	3	3	M. I.	
28	F	75	3	4	Arter. H. D.[e]	Atrial fibrillation. Ileitis
29	M	54	3	2	M. I.	
30	M	57	2.5	3	Claudication	Diab. mell.
31	M	90	3	5	C. V. A.	Arteriosclerotic H. D. Pacemaker
32	F	72	3	6	Arter. H. D.	Atrial fibrillation
33	M	60	2	3	M. I.	
34	M	64	4	4.5	M. I.	Angina pectoris

[a]M. I. = myocardial infarction.
[b]C. V. A. = cerebrovascular accident.
[c]Diab. mell. = diabetes mellitus.
[d]Renal arter. = renal arteriosclerosis.
[e]Arter. H. D. = arteriosclerotic heart disease.

ties in those patients who consume the largest volumes of homogenized milk and milk products. A direct connection exists between the consumption of homogenized milk and levels of BMXO antibodies. This observation was later confirmed and expanded upon by the team of Rzucidlo and Zikakis at the University of Delaware.

The Delaware researchers also conclude that the small quantities of BMXO absorbed over a lifetime "may be biologically very important."

Superoxide

By 1974, the research conducted by Oster and Ross established with reasonable certainty that BMXO was responsible for the depletion of plasmalogen from cardiovascular tissue. For this reason, Oster now felt quite comfortable using the term Plasmalogen Disease, which he had first coined in 1968 to describe the disease process.

With each new finding, BMXO began to loom as one of the major dietary causes of atherosclerosis. Gradually, the puzzle of how plasmalogen disease leads to a heart attack, gangrene, senility, and any of the other health problems of atherosclerosis was pieced together.

After XO finds its way into the artery wall superoxide may be produced. A highly reactive substance, superoxide is employed by the body in its defense against foreign intruders. But in the artery wall superoxide damages plasmalogen. Toxic peroxides, thromboxanes, and potent vasoconstrictors, released by the action of superoxide on the hormone-like prostaglandins may create a toxic biochemical soup for the artery wall.

The lifespan of the active superoxide ion is extremely short, approximately 0.0003 seconds. Another enzyme, superoxide dismutase (SOD), an integral part of the body's intricate system of checks and balances, is responsible for "turning off" superoxide. Without SOD, superoxide would destroy vital structures, such as joint cartilages.

Wherever XO is deposited in the artery wall, superoxide may be created. Oster hypothesizes that SOD may not always be available at the site or, perhaps, it does not arrive at the site in time to neutralize superoxide; the time reference is microseconds. Either one of these possibilities would allow superoxide's damaging effects on cell membranes to be unchecked.

Superoxide forms part of the chain reaction initiated by XO, a reaction which causes a small area of tissue literally to be eaten away.

At the site of arterial injury, increased cell division takes place, a plaque may form, and the body starts the healing process – atherosclerosis!

Blood clots may form adjacent to the plaque. A variety of substances may accumulate, as many as fifteen major natural chemical ingredients including triglycerides, phospholipids, and various minerals such as calcium. The proteins collagen and fibrin are also deposited. Eventually, even cholesterol may become involved.

Gradually, the thickening of the artery wall impairs the circulation of blood and the heart is forced to work harder. This not only increases the risk of a heart attack but also weakens the entire body predisposing a person to a variety of diseases.

The medical community has succeeded in identifying the clinical signs and symptoms of atherosclerosis. However, despite decades of research and vast expenditures of money, the causes of atherosclerosis have eluded researchers.

Oster's research has succeeded in finding a cause. The process seems to begin in youth when the greatest amount of milk is consumed. One last major hurdle still remained. He would have to find a solution, a means for preventing the onset and possibly the progression of the disease process of atherosclerosis.

Decades of Scientific Sleuthing

Nurse O'Neill put the papers down carefully on her desk and turned to look out of the office window. From her thoughtful air, it was clear something was puzzling her.

"Caught you napping, Barbara?"

Oster's voice was amused. He had worked enough years, nearly twenty now, with Barbara O'Neill to know two things with absolute certainty. She was one of the most energetic people he had ever had an opportunity to work with, and she could no more sleep at her desk than she could leap tall buildings at a single bound.

"Doctor, I want you to look at these numbers."

Barbara turned around.

"The lab reports on Mr. and Mrs. D'Amato just came back."

It was obvious that Oster didn't recognize the name, so the nurse added, by way of explanation.

"The young Italian couple we used in the double blind study a few years ago, in 1974, on immune response. We assigned D'Amato as the fictitous name for the couple to preserve anonymity. They were in at the beginning of the week for routine blood tests."

"And?" Oster picked up the lab papers and studied them.

"Both pretty medium, middle of the road results," he said. "What's on your mind?"

"You have the original data from the study in your paper. I'm almost certain the lab reports to-

day show an increase in their antibody levels a-
gainst XO."

Comprehension appeared in the physician's
eyes.

"Now I follow you," he exclaimed. "When we
were compiling the data from the results of the
study, we both remarked on the fact that these two
young people had low antibody responses. Both had
only been in the United States a short time. Do
you remember we suspected this might have been a
significant factor."

"Look at the difference, a few years later. The
figures have definitely increased."

The nurse's voice was emphatic.

"Doctor, please, check on all of the original
figures when you look up the records at home. You
know," she continued, "I distinctly remember asking both of them about the food they ate when they
were growing up in Italy. No junk food, that's certain. I believe the wife had never had any dairy
products except raw goat's milk and some cheese.

"Bride and groom! Sure, I remember them
well," Oster added, pleased with his memory recall.
"They came in for their premarital blood tests and
you enlisted them in the double blind study."

"You singled out the D'Amatos as well as that
young Indian couple for particular discussion," added O'Neill.

Oster turned and headed for his office where
he knew he had a reprint of the original report.
Preoccupied in thought the nurse followed him
down the corridor. If she was correct, her observation could prove significant.

One of the bookcases in the physician's office
was filled exclusively with the scientific papers he
had published. All its shelves bulged with stacks of
papers and bound reports. But, without any hesita-
tion, Oster pulled out a handful of pamphlets from

the second shelf and turned to wave them triumphantly at Barbara O'Neill.

"Here we are, here are the reprints. Published in August 1974, in *American Laboratory*. Our double blind study of people's immune response to XO in cow's milk."

"Let's see, we had a total of seventy-five people in the test group," Oster commented as he skimmed over the report.

Barbara remembered the numbers vividly. This particular study had been her introduction to the fine details of medical detective work. It was the first time she'd had the responsibility for handling the procedure for a double blind test.

"Take this copy."

Oster handed the nurse an extra reprint.

"Good memory, considering it's been several years since we worked on this study. The information on the D'Amatos is in the first column here under 'results'."

Barbara scanned the paragraphs. Oster spotted the material they were searching for first and read it out loud.

"Scrutiny of a few individual cases reveals some interesting observations. Two young healthy Italian immigrants appeared for a required premarital blood test. Both had only +1 agglutination. Their milk history revealed that the 24-year-old bride had been drinking only goat's milk most of her life, and the groom, a country boy, had been given only raw unrefrigerated cow's milk."

"That's it." Her voice was triumphant.

"Here...look, Doctor, you can see their lab results today show a change, a significant increase in the antibody response to XO. They've been in this country several years, and since you don't usually find either goat's milk or raw unrefrigerated cow's milk in the supermarket, undoubtedly they've been drinking homogenized cow's milk." Barbara looked over the next few paragraphs of the report.

"When we did the study back in 1974, do you remember there was also a young couple from India? I believe you also made reference to them in the paper because of the significant difference in XO antibody between the husband and the wife?" she asked the doctor. "They couldn't have had a wider variation. Here it is. The husband, who was 29 years old, had a +1 response, one of the lowest possible, but his 22-year-old wife had a +5 response, the highest possible."

"Good point," Oster responded. He ran his finger down the line of numbers in one of the charts in the paper.

"I see here that when they lived in India, they both drank boiled buffalo milk but after they came to America, the wife started consuming large quantities of homogenized cow's milk, as part of the treatment for her chronic gastroenteritis."

"I wonder if we'd find an increase in the husband's antibody reaction to XO now?"

"I'm sure we'd uncover quite a few interesting details if we updated the responses of the patients in that study," Oster replied. "But the nuts and bolts of the theory are in place." He smiled broadly at Nurse O'Neill.

"If, as some critics suggest, XO in milk is digested and rendered inactive in the stomach, how could anyone have antibodies to it?" Oster asked, rhetorically.

"Come on, Barbara, it's time to close up shop. You're going to deprive me of my daily exercise. Swimming pool hours are over at six-thirty!"

The next day Nurse O'Neill looked up when she heard the outer door to Oster's office click shut. It was well past the time for the day's first appointment; that usually meant one thing, hospitalized patients with problems.

"Morning," Oster's voice, faint at first, became more audible as he crossed the office to hang up his coat.

The nurse hurried down the corridor to the physician's office.

"The waiting room's crowded."

She looked at her wristwatch.

"Hospital rounds took you longer than expected?"

"I was called in at four this morning. Only finished just a few minutes ago. Mrs. Fallner went into the intensive care unit during the night; had a relapse. John Raymond's back with his second myocardial infarct."

The nurse nodded, her face grim.

"We've two emergency visitors on top of the patients already scheduled. One is new. He'd been seeing Doctor Murphy. His name is Charles Snyder, he's a top lawyer from New Haven. He came fully prepared with his records."

Oster looked at the nurse expectantly.

"Why did Doctor Murphy recommend him to me?"

"Snyder came of his own accord. He's been to two university medical centers and quite a few physicians."

"The problem?"

"Nonhealing foot ulcer. He's in severe pain most of the time; can hardly walk. I went over the records he brought. He's been given just about every drug imaginable."

Oster sighed.

"I think I know why he came," he said. "Nonhealing ulcer of the foot? Murphy probably suggested the last resort, amputation. Correct?"

Nurse O'Neill nodded.

"Treatment, Barbara. That's what we need."

As Oster turned back into his office, bracing himself for the work ahead, he thought to himself.

"Until my research produces some sort of reliable treatment, some solution to the problems of atherosclerosis, my work is not complete."

Folic Acid Therapy For XO-engendered Atherosclerosis

"As a longtime opera buff, I'm fond of many different operas, one of which is Kurt Weill's and Bertolt Brecht's wonderful *Threepenny Opera*. In it there is a saying which I've found to be quite true. It goes something like this: 'Make yourself a plan, be a bigshot, then make yourself a second plan. Both will go to naught'."

Great material success or overwhelming official recognition from medical peers may not have come Kurt Oster's way, yet he is anything but a cynic. During his lifetime he has seen his work help many. His satisfaction and success come from the knowledge that so many people with crippling illnesses, including atherosclerosis, have been helped back to active lives by his therapy for XO-engendered atherosclerosis.

Oster's discovery of a treatment for XO-engendered atherosclerosis did not happen the way such accomplishments are often envisioned by Hollywood screen writers. Oster did not stumble upon the solution after mixing chemical upon chemical in a hit or miss fashion until formula #1001 was concocted. The discovery process lacked much of the drama that surrounded his earlier work on the isolation of XO as a culprit. In this instance all Oster needed was his knowledge of applied chemistry and pharmacology, plus a little deductive reasoning, to derive a therapy. The process involved little more than knowing which textbooks to open. However, when Oster first prescribed his treatment in 1970 there was a hitch.

Plasmalogen Disease Therapy

"At first, when I came up with an antidote to the health problems caused by plasmalogen depletion in arteries, I worked with the only known xanthine oxidase inhibitor, the synthetic drug, allopurinol. Although the results were impressive, I was concerned about possible side effects. Allopurinol is very potent, and I suspected it might have serious side effects, especially after prolonged use. I desperately wanted to avoid further complications for my patients. Remember, we're talking about the treatment of people who already have major health problems. As a physician, and as someone who's suffered two heart attacks, I knew that adding a powerful drug like allopurinol to the situation might not be in the patient's best interests.

"I again checked the scientific literature and found that folic acid, a natural B vitamin, was described as an inhibitor of xanthine oxidase. The theoretical basis by which folic acid inhibits XO was first described in the 1940s by the celebrated Danish biochemist Herman Kalckar, who did this work at Harvard University.

"Like all vitamins, folic acid has a multiplicity of functions in the body. It is essential for blood cell formation and, therefore, prevents certain types of anemias. It is essential for DNA and RNA synthesis in all cells. It also participates in the synthesis of choline which is needed for plasmalogen formation. A folic acid deficiency also hinders the formation of antibodies by the immune system.

"In essence, the benefits of folic acid have long been known, but I've never found any reference in the medical literature to show it has been used for any therapeutic purpose other than correcting vitamin deficiencies and certain anemias. Large pharmaceutical manufacturers cannot expect to profit from the manufacture and marketing of folic acid because it is not possible to patent folic acid. Look at the problems we're having treating patients with rare diseases because manufacturers are reluctant to produce the so-called orphan drugs. They provide known benefits but no profits.

"Our first task, once we decided to use folic acid, was to arrive at an appropriate dosage. I should point out that because of our habit of referring to the treatment as folic acid therapy, people don't realize the tablets also contain ascorbic acid, or vitamin C, to help the intestinal absorption of folic acid. A person can take all the folic acid he wants, but unless it is absorbed, the body cannot utilize it. Think of it like this. You have a bottle of medicine in your pocket but if you can't get the bottle open, the medicine won't be of any use.

"More specifically, in order for the body to make use of folic acid, vitamin C is combined with it, in equal proportions, to activate intestinal enzymes, dihydrofolate transferase in particular, necessary for optimal absorption of folic acid. Chemically, folic acid is most active in its reduced form, tetrahydrofolic acid. To maintain this reduced state and to prolong shelflife by preventing folic acid from being oxidized, I added ascorbic acid which is a natural antioxidant. Nature usually offers us the ideal combinations of the two vitamins in foods. Man's primary sources of folic acid include leafy greens, asparagus, lentils, liver, and kidney.

"The dietary intake of folic acid, in the average person, is approximately 300 micrograms (mcg.) per day, even though 400 mcg. is the recommended dietary allowance. If a person has XO-engendered atherosclerosis, our calculations indicate that the therapeutic dosage necessary for folic acid to inhibit XO is about 80 milligrams. Because each person does not absorb folic acid from the gut with the same efficiency, blood levels are checked to make sure patients maintain a blood level of 200 ng per 100 ml after abstaining from folic acid for 12 hours. The oral dosage of 80 mg is 200 times the average daily amount supplied to a person through the diet.

"It should be understood that although folic acid and vitamin C are safe, over-the-counter supplements, we do not advocate self-therapy without the supervision of a physician. We start treatment only after a patient's blood test reveals the presence of high levels of antibody to XO. Once a person is on this therapy, vitamin B_{12} levels must be monitored and repleted accordingly since a high intake of folic acid may mask pernicious anemia which is a symptom of a more serious condition affecting the spinal column due to a B_{12} deficiency. Clinically, pernicious anemia is characterized by fatigue and by enlarged red blood cells. Known as a 'combined system disease,' the disease can be corrected by vitamin B_{12}. Folic acid, while masking the symptoms, does not prevent irreversible damage to nerve tissue while B_{12} does.

"When we started with the therapy, I was one of the first to try it: I had so little to lose and everything to gain."

At his desk, cheerfully coping with the constant demands of his busy day, Oster keeps up with an endless flow of data concerning the progress of his patients on folic acid therapy.

"I find that patients frequently recommend the treatment to relatives and friends who have similar circulatory problems." He nods, pleased by this fact; the highest recognition any therapy can be accorded.

"The results have been truly remarkable. I'm a good example of what happens when someone with atherosclerosis which may have been caused by XO starts folic acid therapy. I've been taking what the FDA calls pharmacologic doses of folic acid since the early 1970s. Excellent results, no significant adverse side-effects for over twelve years now.

"Before I started taking folic acid, I required about six nitroglycerine tablets a *day* to relieve chest pains. I was literally forced to use nitro to get through the day without severe pain. Now, I'm down to about zero to three nitro tablets a *week*. A substantial difference! I'm on the therapeutic dose of folic acid, down from eighty to forty milligrams daily. That is, I take one twenty milligram tablet in the morning, one more in the evening. Ross and I discovered through our laboratory study that anything less than forty milligrams a day may not be effective in inhibiting XO-engendered atherosclerosis. Ross is also now using folic acid because when he checked his blood for antibodies to XO, he showed the high antibody level of +4.

"Unfortunately, as of 1971, a physician in the United States needs a special license from the Food and Drug Administration, called an Investigator's New Drug Application, in order to prescribe dosages larger than 1 mg tablets of folic acid. And, the limitations on buying folic acid over-the-counter are even more restrictive.

"It's truly baffling that folic acid is the vitamin singled out by the FDA for this type of ban, particularly when no toxic side effects have ever been reported from its use. Based on the results of several hundred patients whom I have treated, I can see no problems with therapeutic doses of folic acid. It is by far the best therapy I know for retarding the progression of XO-engendered atherosclerosis.

"I would like to emphasize the fact that my personal reaction to this therapy has been excellent. Almost every year, I travel abroad. I take strenuous trips and lecture in other parts of the world: China, Africa, and Europe. For a 74-year-old I lead an active life. I suspect it is folic acid therapy that makes it possible.

"Most people I know who have had two heart attacks, as I had, along with ensuing angina, are forced into a sedentary existence, even with the best of the accepted drug medications. These unfortunate people are told by their physicians to face reality and are advised that they must resign themselves to a life devoid of most of its pleasures. No exertion, no strenuous activity, no cholesterol...the list is quite extensive. There's no doubt the folic acid-ascorbic acid therapy has given me a new lease on life. Most of my patients feel the same way. I'll cite a few case histories. Of course, I won't use the actual names of these patients out of respect for their privacy. The results are most positive, some may say miraculous. They deserve to receive attention."

Case Histories

"I still have records of treatment with allopurinol, the synthetic drug I tried at the very beginning of our investigation. I had to use the same large doses of this drug as ordinarily prescribed in the treatment of gout, where it is used to inhibit XO in the liver. But, as I have already pointed out, allopurinol may produce serious drawbacks when used in the required massive doses over a long period of time. During the time I prescribed allopurinol, the results were excellent because allopurinol and folic acid work in the same way: each is known to inhibit XO."

CASE A
Climbing Stairs Again

"Someone whom I'll call Mrs. A, a woman in her fifties, originally came to me with crippling angina. I treated her for years with cholesterol-reducing drugs, yet she remained disabled to the point where she could not handle light housework. Her husband had to do it. Her chest pains also came at night and were only endured with the help of nitroglycerine tablets kept at hand on the bedside table. What a way to live!

"Mrs. A was taking fifteen nitro tablets every 24 hours. A high dosage. At first, I started Mrs. A with small 100 mg doses of allopurinol, but her condition did not improve. Every two weeks the allopurinol dosage was increased until finally, the magic number was reached and Mrs. A experienced dramatic relief. She telephoned my office to report that for the first time in years she had gone through a night without serious angina pain. Within days, Mrs. A found she could start living like everyone else. She could go upstairs, she could do the housework, she could look after herself. She could even go out by herself. In other words, Mrs. A could enjoy a normal life again.

"When I reported this result to the people over at Burroughs Wellcome and Co., the firm that manufactures allopurinol, they suggested that the only way to prove the drug was responsible for producing the positive results was for me to do a double blind test. Mrs. A agreed to participate in the experiment.

"After the experiment was started Mrs. A soon called me up to say the medication no longer seemed to be effective and that the chest pains were coming back. Not knowing whether she was receiving the placebo or the drug, the only thing I could do aside from terminate the test was to tell her to give the pills a chance, but from what she told me I began to suspect she was on the placebo. Then, misfortune struck. Mrs. A, while attempting to walk up her stairs went into cardiac failure and was rushed to Yale Medical Center where she died of irreversible congestive heart failure. After this I broke the double blind code and found out she had indeed been on placebo. Ever since I have refused to perform double blind tests even though they could help substantiate my work with XO-engendered atherosclerosis."

CASE B
Active Again After Two Heart Attacks

"One of the very first patients I started on therapeutic doses of folic acid came to me after her physician retired and moved away. I'll call her Mrs. B. She'd suffered two severe heart attacks which had left her with disabling chest pains. When she first arrived in my office, I sent her to the lab for the antibody test to establish the extent to which her arteries may have been exposed to XO and to establish whether folic acid therapy was needed. Mrs. B's antibody level turned out to be very high. I, therefore, prescribed therapeutic doses of folic acid.

"Mrs. B walks every day with her husband, near their house, where there's a small hill. Mrs. B always had to take nitro, either before or after climbing the hill, to combat the chest pains caused by this exertion. Within weeks of beginning folic acid therapy, she could climb the hill without having chest pains. Not only that, but her need for nitro diminished dramatically.

"Mrs. B just couldn't understand the change.

"In her case XO-induced plasmalogen depletion may have led to two heart attacks. Folic acid blocked the process and may have helped restore plasmalogen in her arteries. I wish I could say the disease was permanently halted. I can't. We've found circulating antibodies to XO in elderly patients years after they have stopped drinking homogenized milk and years after they have been taking therapeutic doses of folic acid. That's why it seems to be necessary to maintain the dosage on a daily basis. Once deposited in the cardiovascular tissues, XO doesn't seem to go away, and certain factors may enhance its activity. Folic acid may counterbalance these factors.

"Like most patients, Mrs. B isn't concerned with how the therapy works. She's simply very happy to be living life free of pain and the restraints atherosclerosis often imposes. Now she continues to work full time and can walk out of her home with her husband and confidently climb the hill, knowing that somehow folic acid is helping her."

CASE C
Instead of Bypass Surgery

"Another one of my early patients was someone I'll call Mr. C, although he's actually a bishop of his church, so I suppose it would be more appropriate to refer to him as Bishop C. Ever since I started prescribing folic acid therapy Bishop C has enjoyed an active, normal life. He came to see me because he had been told that if he didn't have a bypass operation within three months his life would be in jeopardy.

"Need I say that Bishop C has never had the operation because he opted to take folic acid instead.

"In this case I also started with an antibody test. His level was high, so we started therapy. Since that time, almost ten years ago, he's led a perfectly normal life."

CASE D
A Cardiac Cripple

"Another patient, Mr. D, a man in his fifties, came to me after he'd had one heart attack and a pulmonary embolism. The poor fellow was a cardiac cripple. He was also on a disability pension. I went through the routine diagnostic procedures and then prescribed the therapeutic dose of folic acid. He responded very well and started to again lead an active life. However, Mr. D once ran out of folic acid and, sure enough, two weeks later had another heart attack. Mr. D survived the second heart attack, but some time later, while working at home, he suffered a second pulmonary embolism. He was taken to Park City Hospital. The newly appointed chairman of the institutional review committee at the hospital was an adamant supporter of the cholesterol and saturated fat dogma and consequently did not understand how folic acid therapy could benefit a patient. In fact, he forbid the hospital staff to provide Mr. D with folic acid. Mr. D had to furnish his own folic acid which his relatives brought to him. While the nurses watched with great trepidation, he took his folic acid. Mr. D recovered, and for the past ten years he has been conscientious about not running out of folic acid.

"An interesting twist to the story is that the hospital director who forbade the use of folic acid himself had a heart attack and subsequent bypass surgery. Would you believe he is still not disillusioned with the cholesterol theory?"

CASE E
Most Dramatic Result

"I have had tremendous results with patients who have peripheral artery disease accompanied by gangrene. Mr. E who was a diabetic and an inveterate smoker developed threatening gangrene in his big toe. It became discolored and was extremely painful. He had no evidence of infection. On 80 mg of folic acid per day the condition was reversed in just two weeks; a condition which with all other known medications usually progresses to infection and amputation. I might add that the gangrene disappeared despite Mr. E's refusal to give up smoking as he was advised."

Believing the Results

"All the cases I've handled help substantiate the theoretical aspects of my work. Granted, not every pathway in the arterial XO-disease process has been explained, but at least we have established one factor that may trigger atherosclerosis and how we may negate this factor. I am convinced that the folic acid therapy, if used when appropriate, would help an overwhelming percentage of the millions who have symptoms of atherosclerosis initiated by XO."

Oster is apprehensive about discussing with his peers the hundreds of case histories of patients who have benefited from therapeutic doses of folic acid. He is very conscious of the fact that the medical profession often terms this type of reporting testimonial or anecdotal because it's not a substitute for double blind clinical trials.

As much as Oster sympathizes with the opinion of his medical peers about the value of double blind testing, he explains it is not a reasonable demand.

"It's true that without double blind testing, no one can prove that therapeutic doses of folic acid have definitely been responsible for the positive results. However, let me remind you that before a therapy is approved, double blind testing is not always necessary. Coronary bypass surgery, in which a vein is taken from the leg and used to reroute blood flow past an obstruction in the coronary artery, is a prime example. In response to criticism that I haven't proven the therapy with double blind methods, I reiterate that no physician, anywhere, is willing to assume the responsibility of testing drugs by double blind methods when the cases are life-threatening. This means we may never be able to prove conclusively that our successes are the result of folic acid administration.

"Our results, however, speak for themselves. Unfortunately, they are largely ignored by the medical community. The why doesn't concern me. Historically, innovation has been ignored, even shunned. However, certain practical aspects do concern me, most particularly the fact that so many millions of people who may benefit from this therapy are not receiving it. The objections could be silenced with a comprehensive clinical trial with patients who have atherosclerosis due to XO. This may be the only way to convince the medical community.

"Consider these several points. My case histories are documented over a number of years. We have case after case in which formerly crippled individuals with atherosclerosis have actually been able to start leading normal lives. That is very uncommon in the practice of cardiology. As far as I know, we have accomplished a great deal more than anyone else has with any other medication.

"The initial lesion which leads to atherosclerosis obviously may be caused by more than one factor, so we need more than one answer. I, however, have concentrated my research on the specific area of plasmalogen depletion in arteries. Folic acid therapy seems to be a viable way for combating one cause of atherosclerosis."

Charting Reactions

In 1971, Oster designed a chart summarizing the consequences of plasmalogen depletion by XO. The chart "Plasmalogen Disease Manifestation," shows four possible categories of damage. According to the diagram below, plasmalogen depletion in the arterial wall may result in atherosclerosis. If this depletion takes place in the heart muscle, it may lead to myocardial infarction, scarring, and possibly irregular heart beat. In the myelin sheath

Figure 4.

PLASMALOGEN DISEASE MANIFESTATION

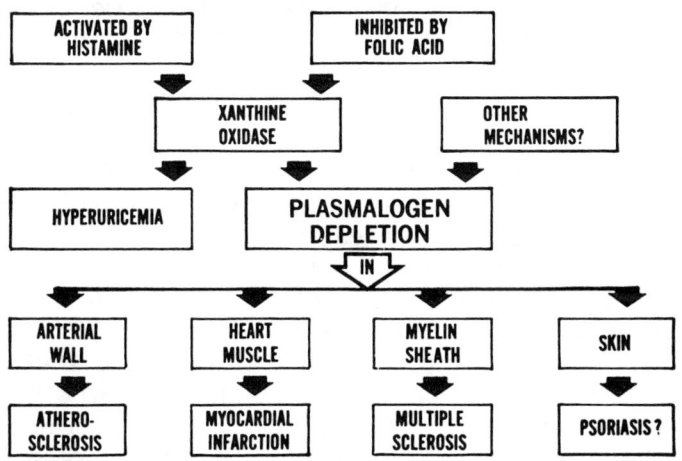

© 1971 KURT A. OSTER M.D.

of nerve fibers, plasmalogen depletion may contribute to the degeneration of the fatty insulating coat and may represent one initial cause of multiple sclerosis. In the skin, lack of plasmalogen may lead to psoriasis."

Oster, referring to the chart explains:

"You'll notice that one of the boxes on the chart raises the query 'other mechanisms?' I must stress here, again, that there's little doubt atherosclerosis has *more than one cause.* My research has uncovered *one* of the dietary causes. In any case, the health problems listed in this chart are significant and should be investigated thoroughly. It's worth repeating that the consequences of atherosclerosis are varied and serious. Whether we're talking of mental problems, stroke, gangrene, aneurisms, kidney disease, myocardial infarction or angina pectoris — even abdominal angina, which is pain caused by an insufficient blood supply to the intestines — it's important to remember that atherosclerosis lies behind such illnesses.

"The traditional methods treat symptoms. And, they involve either expensive synthetic drugs, with their often attendant serious side effects, or procedures such as balloon compression of lesions, or surgical bypass. Such procedures continue to escalate medical costs in the United States while doing little to stem the tide of atherosclerosis because all too frequently, symptoms and not the cause of a disease are treated.

"Few people are aware that after a coronary bypass not everyone can return to work, particularly blue-collar workers whose jobs demand physical activity. Another little-noted fact is that 2 percent of more than 100,000 Americans who had such surgery in 1981 did not survive this operation and that in another 10 percent the grafted vessels closed up within a year. Unlike surgery, my therapy efficiently zeroes in on one of the more important causes and results are not short-lived."

Scientific Papers

The medical establishment's failure to consider the work of Oster and Ross, in particular the folic acid therapy, is difficult to comprehend. Their reports are well-documented and have been published in some of the most respected medical journals. Oster has published two papers which describe the clinical results of his folic acid therapy. The first, "The Absorption and Inhibition of Xanthine Oxidase," appeared in *American Laboratory*, October 1976. In this report Oster provides the truly remarkable results of the first few years of his successful therapy.

> Sixty patients are at present under study with the combination of folic acid and ascorbic acid. Daily doses of 80 mg of folic acid produced remarkable clinical effects, especially measureable and observable in peripheral arteriosclerosis of diabetic patients.
>
> A 57-year-old diabetic male exhibited a nonhealing foot ulcer of one year's duration, painful, undermined, and partially gangrenous. The ulcer had been treated with all known modalities of potentially effective drugs now obtainable, with negative results. The patient was in continuous pain. He sought medical advice at two major university centers in the country. He underwent arteriographic examinations and was faced with the threat of amputation. He responded dramatically to combined folic and ascorbic acid therapy, with no changes in the diet or in his diabetic control with sulfonylurea. Even cigarette smoking was continued. Three months of daily administration of folic acid and ascorbic acid changed him from a crippled individual, who could not walk 100 yards because of the pain, to one who

could once more perambulate. Five months after the inception of the new treatment, he danced at his son's wedding and proceeded to play nine holes of golf.

Similar heartening results were obtained with eight additional cases, male and female, in the age group of 50-89 years. For this reason, the author has described folic acid in combination with ascorbic acid as the 'penicillin equivalent' for the treatment of amenable atherosclerotic clinical manifestations. The combination has excellent therapeutic effects without damage to the patient – the ideal drug.

The puzzling question of the absorption of xanthine oxidase by the gut has been partially answered by the discovery of specific antibodies against this enzyme in the sera of human patients. Those with atherosclerotic manifestations had a significantly higher antibody titer than those without atherosclerosis. The determination of antibodies to xanthine oxidase may provide a screening method for the presence or absence of atherosclerotic lesions. The experiments with folic acid inhibition of xanthine oxidase in atherosclerotic manifestations are being continued. An illustrative case of peripheral atherosclerotic lesion benefited by the treatment is described in detail.

The second article appeared in March 1981, as a short entry in volume forty of the *Federation of American Societies for Experimental Biology*. It succinctly summarizes the therapy.

ATHEROSCLEROSIS TREATED WITH FOLIC ACID.... Daily doses of 40-80 mg of folic acid (FA) were investigated during nine years in 198 atherosclerotic patients for effectiveness, safety, and eventual side effects. Serum FA levels were monitored. Positive immune reaction to bovine milk xanthine oxidase (BMXO) determined patient suitability. Persorption of BMXO in liposomal form has been proven in both humans and animals. This enzyme, ectopically deposited, depletes a phospholipid component of the cell membrane, plasmalogen. FA prevented myocardial infarction in 25 cases, alleviated angina pectoris, and reduced nitroglycerin needs in 31 cases. FA prevented gangrene in peripheral atherosclerosis in 13 cases. In a non-FA group, no difference in deaths due to pump failure was observed. Five cases of non-fatal myocardial infarction were ascribed to low serum FA levels, in spite of confirmed high intake. A low serum FA in the presence of an elevated red cell folate was discovered during this investigation for the first time. FA has been found to be safe and effective with no untoward reactions in the treatment and prevention of atherosclerotic lesions caused by the persorption of BMXO.

In short, the report describes a simple, safe, and inexpensive treatment for a killer disease. It sounds like news that would bring excited reactions from the medical community.

The 198 patients who were successfully treated by Oster with folic acid were fortunate to have met this medical pioneer. Another physician would have most likely recommended open heart surgery for many of the patients. The alternative folic acid therapy spared many patients bills in the range of $15,000 to $25,000 for invasive surgery and all that such surgery entails – the foot-long scar, the sawed open rib cage, and the bones which are clamped back so as to expose the heart. Bruised bones ache for weeks. Above all, Oster's patients were not exposed to the operation's mortality risk.

Instead of receiving praise or encouragement from the medical community, Oster only received more criticism after his findings were published. He was advised to test folic acid in by using double blind methods.

"Impossible," Oster states. "I've already had one bad experience with this type of testing.

"Now I don't mean it cannot be done. I mean that it would be morally and ethically irresponsible. How could I say to a patient with severe angina pains, here's a tablet which may alleviate your pain; it's helped a lot of people in your situation. But it may be a placebo, an innocent sugar pill, not the real medication.

"In light of my sobering personal experience with one double blind clinical trial I don't see how any physician could consider taking away a patient's nitroglycerine tablets offering the sugar pill instead. Of course not, it's morally wrong. When patients rely on you to help them correct a life-threatening situation, you cannot turn that into an experiment. Angina pains are serious and unpleasant. Gangrene is very serious. You cannot deprive people of a therapy that works because you wish to study it. My responsibility is to do all I can to help them.

"Recent studies investigating hypertension and atherosclerosis have not been employing double blind methods. The studies I'm referring to differentiated only between usual care and experimental care groups.

"There are numerous examples where certain procedures or medications have not had to pass double blind testing before gaining acceptance. A number of drugs presently on the market never underwent double blind testing. As I have stated already, bypass surgery was never subjected to double blind clinical trials. And, I might add that even after a therapeutic measure is put through such tests, there is no automatic guarantee of favorable results.

"I once happened to be one of those unfortunate enough to use a tested and approved drug produced by Smith, Kline, and French called Selacryn. The generic name is ticrynafen, an antihypertensive diuretic, a drug designed to decrease uric acid levels in patients with high blood pressure. However, after I took it I became deathly sick. Some people died after using this double blind tested, FDA-approved medication. The situation with this drug is not unique. Atromid-S (clofibrate), a cholesterol-reducing drug, also had the double blind seal of approval. Yet today it is banned in many countries because it causes gallstones. At one time Atromid-S was the second most prescribed drug in the United States. Today its use is down to a trickle. The blatant advertising by its manufacturer that brainwashed physicians has stopped. However, the blind faith physicians had in the drug reflects poorly on their independent judgements. So much for testing and government approval!"

In contrast to a number of drugs, folic acid is not toxic and is even essential for pregnant women. In the 1950s a physician, L. Peer, did some pioneering work with folic acid deficiencies and their association with cleft palate, a condition in which an infant is born with part of the roof of the mouth cavity missing. Physicans today frequently prescribe daily doses of 1 mg of folic acid to pregnant women to prevent cleft palate in the newborn.

A Virtual Ban
—The FDA Limits Folic Acid Use and Sale

For years, folic acid tablets of various strengths were produced by American pharmaceutical manufacturers for over-the-counter sales, and was also sold on prescription up to 20 mg.

In 1971, however, the FDA severely curtailed over-the-counter sales of folic acid and put a very strict limit on the amount to be prescribed by any physician without a special license. As a result the number of companies manufacturing folic acid has dropped sharply, and the strength of the tablets manufactured is set according to those latest FDA requirements.

The FDA's folic acid dosage limit for over-the-counter sale is 800 micrograms, or 0.8 milligrams. Actually, the limit is really set at 400 micrograms, or 0.4 milligrams, but an exception is made for pregnant or lactating women. They may purchase up to 800 micrograms. As it turns out, no vendor asks customers their reasons for buying the higher dosage, so the ceiling, for all practical purposes, is 0.8 milligrams. This is far short of the dosage required to inhibit XO-engendered atherosclerosis.

A microgram is one-thousandth of a milligram. If the therapeutic dose of folic acid for XO-engendered atherosclerosis is 80 milligrams daily, an individual would need about a hundred of the over-the-counter 800 microgram tablets each day to combat XO. That's an impractical amount of pills for a person to take and most people would not even consider it.

Does a similar ban exist outside of the United States? A survey of other nations reveals the U.S. seems to have the most rigid restrictions on folic acid use of any nation. In Canada folic acid is available over-the-counter in 5 milligram strength tablets. In Germany the use of folic acid has been approved as a viable therapy for psoriasis (something Oster first proposed in the early 1970s). Yet, in the United States even physicians are limited in the dosage they may prescribe unless they obtain a special New Drug Application from the FDA.

During the decades that folic acid was freely available in the United States not one case of adverse or toxic side effects was ever reported when it was used correctly. So why the sudden restrictions? Even with the high dosage used by Oster, in thirteen years there have been no significant toxic side effects due to the low toxicity of folic acid in humans. The same applies to experimental animals, attested to in pharmacology textbooks.

"The FDA has given one specific reason for its ban: folic acid can mask complications of pernicious anemia in humans.

"Is this something that affects most of us? Hardly." Oster shakes his head in amazement at government bureaucracy.

"The FDA took a mini truth and blew it out of proportion. Granted, the rationale for the FDA ban has its own accuracy. The flaw is that it applies to a distinct minority within a minority and even then the potential for any health problem is small. Any competent physician would be able to recognize such a problem."

Today, people with XO-engendered atherosclerosis are being deprived of folic acid because of the FDA's concern that folic acid in high dosages might mask the underlying nerve condition of pernicious anemia. Since this condition affects a small percentage of the population, 0.5 percent of those over the age of 65, and since BMXO-engendered atherosclerosis affects approximately 50 percent of the population, it is clear that the benefits of folic acid outweigh any potential risk.

The FDA has been inconsistent in its actions. Has it put restrictions on the allowable over-the-counter vitamin C dosage because of the remote concern that high vitamin C intake may increase the chance of oxalate kidney stone formation in certain people under certain conditions? No. Have they banned or even restricted over-the-counter sales of sugar-sweetened cough medicine and lozenges because diabetics cannot use them without serious consequences? No. Warnings are placed on the label copy of certain over-the-counter medications citing restrictions that might apply to specific individuals. Why can't the same be done with folic acid in high dosages?

Folic acid therapy is an important achievement. It removes the burden of exorbitant costs that patients face with other treatments because all that is involved is the antibody test and the subsequent tests for monitoring folic acid levels in the blood, along with the cost of the vitamin.

When is a Vitamin a Drug?

Most physicians know little more about vitamins and vitamin therapy than the smattering retained from their basic training. They know a lot more about drugs. And the detail men and women, sales representatives from pharmaceutical manufacturers, flood the offices of physicians with a constant shower of material on the drug products they wish to sell.

Research into vitamin therapy in the 1920s and 1930s, slowed down when antibiotics became available. With the advent in the 1940s of the so-called wonder drugs, such as penicillin and streptomycin, vitamin therapy was first neglected, then scorned. Thanks to antibiotics, such infectious diseases as pneumonia and tuberculosis are no longer claiming lives at an early age, as was common in the first half of the twentieth century. The death rate of newborns before antibiotics was considerable, now it has been reduced. More and more people are living beyond the age of fifty. This is when degenerative diseases all too frequently catch up with people.

Surgery and symptomatic drug treatment are the modalities accepted by orthodox medicine for treating degenerative diseases, while vitamin therapy is still sadly neglected. Medical schools still teach their students that vitamins are to be employed for correcting overt vitamin deficiency diseases. They have neglected to explore the possible use of vitamins to retard or reverse degenerative disease.

Undoubtedly, part of the resistance to Oster's work lies in his use of a vitamin as if it were a drug when most physicians have been told that any vitamin therapy is "near quackery." Even worse, in the folic acid therapy pharmacological doses of a well-known vitamin have achieved what powerful drugs can not do. Oster is not using folic acid to correct a vitamin deficiency. The high vitamin dosage is aimed at saturating tissues to inhibit XO's damage. After the initial, tissue-saturating dose, many patients require only a smaller, maintenance control doses to keep tissues saturated.

A welter of confusion exists over the use of vitamin megadoses for therapy and the need for vitamin supplements for optimal health. Medical practitioners hesitate to become embroiled in the debate over the value of vitamins. Instead they tend to turn unseeing eyes on any therapy that involves the use of a vitamin with the exclusion of megadoses of niacin, another B vitamin, for the reduction of serum cholesterol.

A Practical Protocol

In order to keep his special license from the FDA to prescribe folic acid in amounts larger than those generally allowed since the 1971 restrictions, Oster must send the FDA an update of his work each year.

In December 1980, Oster received a letter from the Director of the FDA's Division of Metabolism and Endocrine Drug Products. In it, the

Director claimed that pharmacologic doses of folic acid over prolonged periods of time cause a deficiency of the intrinsic factor — a substance produced by cells in the stomach lining. This factor must bind to vitamin B_{12} before B_{12} can be absorbed.

"This in itself is quite a gem," Oster remarks. "I've been unable to find and verify this information in any textbook or any medical journal and since I was supplied with no references concerning this finding, it is, in my opinion, a totally unfounded statement. This is not what you hope for or expect from a representative of government. But there is more to the story."

The Director had also apparently misunderstood the reasons for Oster's use of folic acid. Perhaps he hadn't looked over the file carefully. He actually wrote that Oster had stated folic acid could prevent atherosclerosis or coronary heart disease. Oster was astounded by the inaccuracy of the letter.

"From the very beginning, as can be seen from my published works, I've clearly outlined why folic acid therapy is useful. I've stated that my research has shown it serves to inhibit, or help stop, XO-engendered atherosclerosis. And I've clearly stated that the cause of this type of atherosclerosis is the plasmalogen depletion caused by XO in homogenized milk."

"All too frequently, critics of my work make totally unfounded statements and then refuse to offer any reliable references for their objections," Oster explains as he frowns. "The result is objections that seem reasonable but which are actually not accurate. That is why I have agreed to publish my response to that letter from the FDA."   It reads:

...,M.D., Director
Division of Metabolism and Endocrine Drug Products
Bureau of Drugs
Department of Health, Education, and Welfare
Food and Drug Administration
Rockville, Maryland 20857

Dear Dr. ...:

In compliance with your letter of December 18, 1980, I am continuing with the warning on the Folic Acid copy; see sample enclosed. I am also enclosing a Protocol for folic acid studies designed for the use of an IND holder, directed to the Institutional Review Committee of Park City Hospital in Bridgeport.

The data you desire cannot be provided without the necessary financial basis which I am unable to obtain. Nevertheless, I do not think that because of this monetary difficulty, the study should be abandoned, and I am continuing to do the best I can under the circumstances. Even with a half billion dollars spent on the diet-heart problem, the proof of the efficacy of serum cholesterol lowering has not been obtained in spite of randomization of a large number of subjects. Double blinding was also used in the estrogen administration to male patients in the coronary heart studies, and the patients' voices became high pitched, they lost their facial hair, and their mammary glands grew. Who was blind in this instance?

Your fifth paragraph was not clear to me. I would appreciate it if you can send me some documentation for your statement that pharmacological doses of folic acid over prolonged periods of time cause a deficiency of intrinsic factor. I have looked through the publication, FOLIC ACID – BIOCHEMISTRY AND PHYSIOLOGY IN RELATION TO THE THE HUMAN NUTRITION REQUIREMENT of the National Research Council's Food and Nutrition Board of the National Academy of Sciences, (1977) and

through the book, FOLIC ACID IN NEUROLOGY,
PSYCHIATRY, AND INTERNAL MEDICINE, edited
by M. I. Botez, M.D., and E. H. Reynolds, M.D.,
(Raven Press – 1979) and have not found any reference to your statement. Maybe I have overlooked
it and you are aware of something I do not know.
I have talked by telephone to Dr. Neville Coleman
of the State University of New York's Department
of Medicine at Downstate Medical Center in Brooklyn, an outstanding researcher on folic acid. He
assured me that I am doing work in virgin territory
which has never been done and published in the
literature. You have to realize that the study
is now going on for nine and a half years and, so
far, no complication has been discovered.

The question of danger of pernicious anemia vs.
the benefit for atherosclerosis due to bovine milk
xanthine oxidase (BMXO) should be judged in perspective. According to Beeson and McDermott's
TEXTBOOK OF MEDICINE, the incidence of pernicious anemia is one in 200 in patients over 65;
whereas the incidence of atherosclerosis due to
BMXO, from my own personal observation in the
same age group, is at least 50 per cent. According
to your reasoning, you would then deny a beneficial
treatment to 50 per cent of the population in fear
of a potential damage which might occur to one-half
of one per cent.

In your letter, I missed completely any reference
by you to the danger of BMXO contained in liposomes caused by the homogenization of the milk.

You seem to have misunderstood when you say
that I claim efficacy of folic acid for the prevention of atherosclerosis or coronary heart disease.
You seem to have missed the point of our research
completely. It is the Food and Drug Administration's task, according to our research, to begin
to prevent atherosclerosis and coronary heart
disease by providing the American people with
a milk with no biologically available xanthine

oxidase. As long as you do not react to this problem which belongs in your hands, you do not fulfill
your obligation to preserve and guard the health
of the American people.

After all this time, I think I can demand an explanation for your inactivity in this field. If you use
research done in the College of Agriculture of
the University of California at Davis by Ho and
Clifford as an excuse for your inaction, I refer
you to an article in the NEW YORK TIMES of
December 3, 1980, where it states that research
is determined by "Money can influence – or dictate
what research gets done" or "If industry pays the
tab, they've got a right to call the tune."

I hope to receive your answer in the near future.

Sincerely yours,

Kurt A. Oster, M.D.

"I don't hesitate to call a spade a spade," Oster
says. "For all these years, Ross and I have had a
multitude of inaccuracies printed about our work.
Ho and Clifford, sponsored by the Dairy Council,
recently published a critique of our work in the
Journal of Clinical Nutrition. The inacuracies in
this article greatly upset Ross and myself. Their
bias only further exposes their true colors. All
things considered, I think we've been more than patient. We're not interested in political infighting.
We don't rely on grants from industry to support
our work. Our motivation is results."

Oster puts down the copy of his letter to the
FDA and pulls out one of his desk drawers. Holding
up a small brown bottle, he waves it for emphasis.

"Take a look at the label on this. The folic
acid tablets in this bottle are manufactured for me
by MK Laboratories."

The company's name is on the side of the label. The front label reads: folic acid 20 mg, ascorbic acid 20 mg. But it is the left hand side of the

label to which Oster directs attention. The warning printed there is in compliance with FDA regulations:

CAUTION: This amount of folic acid is considered a new drug. Limited by Federal Law to investigational use.

"You can see that I'm not fighting with the FDA's statement, even though Ross and I consider it somewhat unusual. I comply to the utmost with the government's regulations. Every year I have to inform the FDA of my activities, just to bring their file up to date. It's only right that the FDA should know I'm adhering to its rules and regulations. I have no quarrel with doing that. I merely object to inaccurate statements. Remember that my opinion is based on meticulous research and that I, in contrast to some others, try to document my statements and my research.

"I do everything necessary that the FDA rules require. I'd like to see them make changes, of course. But until such changes come, I always have, and always will, comply with regulations.

"I must send the progress of my clinical findings to the FDA so that they know my working methods and results. That's how I keep my special license, the Investigator's New Drug Application (called an INDA in the trade). This FDA license enables me to prescribe folic acid in large doses. Such licenses may be obtained by physicians with the necessary research qualifications if they apply to the FDA," Oster explains.

The FDA requires that the folic acid tablets be manufactured under controlled conditions by an established firm so that high standards are maintained.

Although the entire process of embarking on folic acid therapy is not simple, the steps are fairly straightforward. Qualified physicians can apply to the FDA for the Investigator's New Drug Application to prescribe folic acid. Local labs should be able to test patients' sera for the level of XO antibodies. The remaining steps, if an individual has an antibody reaction between 2 and 5, would be to prescribe folic acid in pharmacological doses. The tablets themselves can be manufactured by drug companies if they have applied for and received the necessary FDA license, the New Drug Application.

Is there a great deal of money to be made from this? Perhaps not at this time, but eventually this might change as the number of consumers using the therapy grows. But there's another consideration.

Responsibility to Profit
— Or the Public Good?

Pharmaceutical manufacturers are business operations committed to showing a profit for their stockholders. They are at the same time in the business of life and death and often have to face the difficult question: where does our responsibility lie, in profit or the public good?

While the drug companies regularly discontinue production of unprofitable drug lines, they observe certain guidelines. These are largely self-imposed by industry; most companies cooperate. By agreement among themselves they take turns in keeping critical, low-sales volume drugs available to the public. Often, the government requests that they do this.

It is not beyond reason to suggest that the formulation of 20 mg of folic acid with 20 mg of vitamin C should eventually become an industry-supported item since its critical need as a control agent for one cause of atherosclerosis has been clearly demonstrated.

If this book does nothing more than encourage part of the medical fraternity, which tacitly endorses Oster's work, to start prescribing folic acid, it will have performed a service.

In all probability, this service may herald the beginning of a new era of treatment for atherosclerosis. The valuable insight the work of Oster and Ross offers may well help other researchers to identify some of the other causes of atherosclerosis.

When he's discussing his work, Oster emphasizes that his forty years of research have had a single result:

"One of the causes of atherosclerosis has been identified."

Although this is a major accomplishment, Oster views it with the dispassionate perspective of the dedicated scientist.

"Still more research is needed to identify what other factors precipitate cardiovascular disease."

A Neglected Prophet

It appears to many of his supporters that Kurt Oster is a neglected prophet.

There is the aphorism: a prophet is not without honor, save in his own country, and in his own house....

Oster's country, his house, has been the medical establishment of the United States.

Despite the meticulous work he has put into research and experimentation to prove atherosclerosis can be initiated by XO, Oster still awaits acceptance by his peers.

Historically, few visionaries in the fields of science and medicine have been recognized in their time. When such visionaries violate the fixed notions of their generation, they very often meet unyielding resistance. The noted physicist, Max Planck, once stated his own experience demonstrates that "a new scientific truth does not triumph by convincing its opponents and making them see the light, but rather because its opponents eventually die and a new generation grows up that is familiar with it."

The reader can help propagate Oster's work; even propagandize it by passing the word to the younger generation. This book can be used as evidence.

The final portion of this book includes some of the key papers that form the body of proof about XO-engendered atherosclerosis and folic acid therapy and should be of interest to most physicians. Many of them are not so much opposed to Oster's work as they are ignorant of it. Open-minded physicians recognize at once the validity of the evidence and the conclusions Oster has drawn.

Oster's papers contain an accumulation of evidence that should convince any objective jury. Once again, one should be reminded that Oster's work has not been accepted by the establishment for one extraordinary reason. No life-and-death, double blind experiments have been performed on human beings. As Oster explains, neither he nor any reputable physician believes in "animal" experiments when the "animals" are human beings and the disease being studied is life-threatening.

"My whole intention with this book is to present a general explanation of the years of research Ross and I have conducted and to offer readers of all backgrounds the opportunity to find out for themselves about XO-engendered atherosclerosis and to know about folic acid therapy.

"Material such as my letter to the FDA is included in this book for one reason only; not to make fun of any mistakes, which may represent a perfectly genuine misunderstanding. Rather, the intention is to help readers understand the attitude Ross and I have to contend with much of the time.

"One of the most commonly asked questions is, 'Why haven't we heard about this therapy?' Although this work is known in my general home area, partly because of newspaper articles and radio broadcasts, outside Connecticut not too many people have heard of XO-engendered atherosclerosis and the therapy.

"Whether objections to the folic-acid therapy are based on mistaken information, or prejudice, or sheer disinterest, one basic fact remains unchanged: our research is accurate. It can be scientifically repeated and has been. People such as Mr. E, who came to me with a non-healing foot ulcer and agreed to try folic acid therapy as a last resort before amputation, had circulation restored in less than three weeks. People with XO-engendered atherosclerosis can be helped. That's the key.

"Each person suffering from atherosclerosis has family or friends who are interested in finding out whether they should be taking folic acid. I'm concerned about helping those whose atherosclerosis is the result of XO – that's a lot of people. My argument isn't with milk, just the homogenization of it.

"I have several wishes. Each is simple.

"First, let's stop homogenizing milk or create a milk free of biologically available XO. Second, let's start helping those with XO-engendered atherosclerosis by removing the restrictions on folic acid."

"At the moment, each of these wishes is frustrated, the first by the milk manufacturers who claim consumers wouldn't like the 'boiled' taste of milk that is ultrapasteurized. The second is frustrated by the FDA's unreasonable limitation of folic acid dosages. I hope that when people come across this book, they'll agree with me and support my objectives. Consumer reaction is most effective in America. It's the consumer who would benefit from my work. I have every hope progress and change will come through them."

Current Treatment Of Atherosclerosis: On The Wrong Track

Oster's twin discovery of one cause of athero-sclerosis and a viable treatment, has met with strong resistance from those intent on maintaining the status quo. Special interest groups have little incentive in seeing popular dogma on atheroslcer-osis displaced. While the FDA – and others – fiddle, Rome burns, and the suffering continues.

In 1981, some thirty million Americans suf-fered some evident form of the painful and debili-tating illness of atherosclerosis. This awesome fig-ure doesn't include people confined to nursing homes or the very large segment of the population whose atherosclerosis goes undetected and undiag-nosed, and therefore untreated.

In one form or another, atherosclerosis claims one million lives in America each year. Cancer, by comparison, is responsible for only a third as many victims. Although atherosclerosis has become the most prevalent disease of the Western world in this century, the magnitude of the effects of athero-sclerosis are deceiving because they are hidden be-hind so many different names: from poor circula-tion to angina pectoris; crippling gangrene to arterial ulceration; strokes, with their paralyzing after effects, to lethal clots; and severe brain damage from ischemia, a condition in which oxygen-rich blood fails to reach organs and tissues.

Few people realize abdominal arteries are also subject to atherosclerosis, the symptoms of which may appear as intestinal angina. Kidneys are often affected, for partial blockage of the renal arteries may lead to renal hypertension.

A Disease of the Young

As extensive as research into atherosclerosis has been, the understanding of the disease by scientists and by the general public has been, and continues to be, fraught with numerous misconceptions.

For many years it was thought that atherosclerosis only occurred in older people since symptoms are rarely obvious in the young. It does not occur to most medical practitioners that their young patients may have the disease. In addition, much of the information about the incidence of the disease in certain age groups has traditionally been obtained from autopsy work. Since relatively few autopsies are performed on children, it was not suspected for many years that atherosclerosis has its antecedents in youth. Over the years, however, it has become increasingly obvious atherosclerosis often starts in infancy.

During the Korean War scientists were shocked to find that young American soldiers killed in combat had "gross evidence of coronary atherosclerosis."

The study revealed a whole range of atherosclerosis, from fatty streaks to fibrous plaques to almost complete narrowing of the coronary arteries. The average age of the 300 soldiers examined was twenty-two. Fourteen of these men had such extensive atherosclerosis that more than one of the main branches of the coronary arteries were 90 percent blocked. There can be little doubt that had these men not been killed in combat, they most certainly would have experienced early death from cardiovascular disease.

Babies who have never indulged in ice cream sundaes, much less had steak for dinner, have been found to have lesions which constitute the initial stage of atherosclerosis called fatty streaks. Such facts helped explode a long-held belief that atherosclerosis is an old person's disease.

Beyond Cholesterol, by M.I.T. neurophysiologists Gruberg and Raymond, challenges the theory that cholesterol in the diet triggers arteriosclerosis and explains that "...pathology reveals that arteriosclerosis, common at all ages, is severe in old people, less severe in adults, and has its antecedents in infants..."

The Many Faces of Atherosclerosis

Whether information is gleaned from autopsies or from symptoms, it is clear that some people can have all of the stages of atherosclerosis at the same time and that the development may go on for years without any clinical symptoms surfacing. Other individuals go from the first to the later stages very rapidly, then suddenly develop a major problem like incapacitating chest pain of angina pectoris, or even heart attacks.

Robert I. Levy, former head of the National Heart, Lung, and Blood Institute explains, "It is a terrible frustration that in about a quarter of heart attack victims, the first clinical sign of atherosclerosis is also the last and terminates in death."

Heart surgeon Michael DeBakey has stated that, "throughout the Western world, and now even in Russia..., heart disease has become the most common cause of death, accounting for more deaths than all other diseases combined." DeBakey adds:

> The commonly used term heart disease is so ill defined and all-encompassing as to be confusing, misleading, and too often, unnecessarily alarming.   Actually, many different types of diseases of the heart and blood vessels are included in the medical term cardiovascular disease. And more than three-fourths of all kinds of heart disease are diseases of the major arteries not of the heart. They are generally due to atherosclerosis....

Proliferation of an Ancient Disease

Another common misconception that continues to prevail, even in professional circles, is that atherosclerosis has always existed on the same scale as it exists today.

Statistics reveal this is not so; the incidence of atherosclerosis skyrocketed in the United States during the late 1930s and early 1940s about the time the practice of homogenization of milk became widespread.

While the epidemic is new, the human race has always been plagued to a lesser degree by atherosclerosis.   Clear medical descriptions of the disease date from the sixteenth century. The English physician Ruffer, investigating the arteries of Egyptian mummies in 1910 found a generous amount "of the disease." He summarized, "There can be no doubt respecting the calcification of the arteries.... The small patches seen in the arteries are atheromatous...lesions are still recognizable...."

The Egyptian mummies were 3,000 years old at the time of the autopsy. This evidence clearly suggests other agents, besides XO, contribute to atherogenesis.

At What Price This Pain?

The current cost of attempting to alleviate the symptoms of atherosclerosis in the United States is staggering. In July 1981, *Time* reported a figure of $50 billion a year, a disturbing increase from the $40 billion recorded during the 1977 Senate hearing on what they called a "killer disease!" By comparison, in the late 1960s figures gathered by the National Heart, Lung, and Blood Institute showed costs were only $15.6 billion per year.

Half of the 1981 $50 billion price tag was for the direct cost of medical care. The balance of the figure consisted of lost wages and productivity, especially noticeable for those in blue collar work who often could not return to full time employment because of physical impairments caused by atherosclerosis.

As of March 1982, coronary bypass surgery was estimated to be a $3.3 billion a year industry. At the beginning of the 1970s, such surgery was considered experimental. In 1982, treatment of heart disease had climbed to $39 billion with lost wages and productivity costs paralleling this increase. Modern civilization is confronted with a very expensive epidemic of atherosclerosis. In ever increasing numbers, atherosclerosis cuts down both the professional and the hardhat with cold impartiality. What is the medical establishment doing to halt the epidemic?

Treating the Symptoms

Although the medical world has defined atherosclerosis as a general disease that affects the whole body, it insists on treating symptoms in different parts of the body separately.

This approach of overlooking cause and of treating only the symptoms of a disease, the tip of the iceberg, is not unique to atherosclerosis. By taking this approach, specialists create, as Betty Friedan writes in a February 1983 article in the *New York Times* magazine, a patient who becomes "a specimen of isolated symptoms."

Research into atherosclerosis is also neatly divided among the locations in which symptoms may surface. Researchers have carefully separated work on the coronary arteries, the brain arteries, the leg arteries, and other peripheral arteries.

What is the result of this convenient division? The *common underlying cause of atherosclerosis* is overlooked, and drugs, surgery, and other treatments are developed for isolated symptoms.

Drugs such as vasodilators, which are designed to improve circulation in the peripheral arteries, and beta blockers, which aid coronary artery circulation, may have some temporary value for the patient. Coronary bypass surgery and the mechanical heart are thought by some to represent supreme advances. New microscope optics and precision microinstruments enable neurosurgeons to restore life-giving circulation to the brains of stroke victims. To accomplish this, neurosurgeons sew together arteries as thin as pencil lead with microsuture, one fifth the thickness of a human hair.

As revolutionary as certain drugs and surgical technologies have become, the underlying factors that initiate atherosclerosis have not been identified. Any health benefits for patients, as a result of drugs or surgery, are often short-lived. As hi-tech as these procedures may appear in color on prime-time television, and as heroic as the surgeons may appear to be, they only generate the illusion of progress, because, in reality, their procedures only serve to slow the progress of ongoing diseases and not stop them. Such treatments are belated efforts to cope, not prevent.

"The sad fact is that most doctors don't realize that preventive medicine is a recognized, board-certified specialty today," laments a specialist in *Physician's Management* magazine. When the same magazine surveyed physicians for its article, "Is Preventive Medicine Really Possible?" a third of the physicians questioned responded that they doubted preventive medicine was practical because of time and cost.

Whose time?

Whose cost?

If a patient is persuaded by his physician to stop smoking (a form of preventive medicine), who saves today's cost of $50,000 to $75,000 for a lung removal with its attendant aftercare? Who saves on the $20,000 (plus) cost of a coronary bypass operation?

In 1981, it was reported that over 2 percent of the 100,000 Americans who had bypass surgery did not survive the operation. In another 10 percent of the patients, the grafted vessels closed up within a year.

In reality, the price tag of preventive medicine comes nowhere close in cost to that of the symptomatic disease care system.

Nonetheless, the debate rages on in the halls of medical institutions...in the schools...in the hospitals...in the research establishments, and, in no area of medicine is the debate more wide-ranging in its applications than in the current approach of modern medicine in dealing with atherosclerosis.

Although many physicians, both general practitioners and specialists, may espouse the idea of preventive medicine – even recognize that it is vital – they face a serious dilemma: what can they do to reverse atherosclerosis once the disease has progressed beyond the point where preventive measures can be taken? What course of treatment should they prescribe for atherosclerosis sufferers? Are bypass operations the solution?

Cardiologists are challenged with such crucial questions concerning life and death daily, in their offices, and hospitals, a probably on the golf course and at dinner parties.

Not an Inherited Disease

Although victims of atherosclerosis have been diagnosed on every continent, it is equally true that not all populations have the same level of susceptibility to the affliction.

"A population group which moves to a new country develops atherosclerosis at a rate which matches that of the local population. You find vastly differing rates of atherosclerosis between the old home and the new country," Oster explains. Japan and Israel exemplify this curious dichotomy.

The results of autopsies on two groups of Japanese between the ages of 50-69 showed striking differences in the rate of atherosclerosis. The first group died in Japan, the second, in Hawaii. Of the Japanese who had remained in their native country, 10 percent had severe atherosclerosis. The figure escalated to 30 percent for the Japanese who had migrated to Hawaii.

The population of Israel is made up of exceedingly diverse ethnic groups. When researchers studied people in one age group, autopsies showed that those who had resided in Israel for the longest period of time had a much higher incidence of atherosclerosis than did recent arrivals.

Epidemiologists investigating atherosclerosis have discovered an interesting link between migrant groups.

Research showed that most migrants developed atherosclerosis at a higher rate, one which paralleled that of the inhabitants in locations to which they had moved.

It has been that way for newcomers to the United States, regardless of where they originally moved from. It also happened to Japanese who moved to Hawaii. Eskimos who went to live in the Hudson Bay area showed the same development of atherosclerosis. People who moved to Israel, the Yemenite Jews from Arabian countries and Ashkenazi Jews from Europe, all developed atherosclerosis at a higher rate.

Evidence such as this ruled out the possibility that genes could play the dominant role in an individual's vulnerability to atherosclerosis. This knowledge was helpful to Oster in the development of his theory.

Since genes do not predispose an individual to the disease, diet must have been the factor in new homelands that increased the susceptibility of some migrants to atherosclerosis.

A Dietary Cause

Thus, Oster's logical examination of cause and effect pointed to the existence of some agent in food that triggered the atheroslcerotic process.

Oster's thinking paralleled that of several other leading researchers, including that of Ancel B. Keys. After comparing the incidence of atherosclerosis in immigrant groups in the United States to the disease frequency in populations in Europe from where the migrants had come, Keys concluded that some dietary factor, which he labeled

"Factor X," is responsible for increasing the prevalence of the disease in the United States by
about 50 percent.

Oster eventually found evidence from an assortment of seemingly unrelated clues to support
his contention that a specific dietary factor is a
culprit in starting the atherosclerotic process.

Hormonal differences between men and wom-
en provided one of the earlier clues.

It has been established that five times as many
men as women between the ages of forty and for-
ty-nine suffer from the primary manifestation of
atherosclerosis: heart attack. Above the age of fifty the ratio in the favor of women begins to decrease.

More specifically, women of premenopausal
age have a much lower heart attack rate than men
of a similar age. Women are clearly less vulnerable
to this health problem than are men until women
reach menopause.

"Why," Oster initially questioned, "is this so?"

Women and men, after all, eat practically the
same foods. How could something in food harm
men but not women? Could some factor in the physical makeup of women protect them?

Since the hormonal balance is the basic difference between the sexes, Oster wondered whether
female hormones may protect women from atherosclerosis and heart attacks. Proving this would be
another matter; it would not be easy.

Gradually the pieces in the puzzle began to
fall into place and the connection between diet and
atherosclerosis became clear.

Oster's search of the medical literature uncovered the work of biochemist G.G. Roussos of the
National Institutes of Health (formerly of Roosevelt
University, in Chicago). Roussos was interested in
the question of why more men than women, by the

factor of 20, suffered from gout, the extremely painful affliction of the joints.

Roussos had painstakingly designed experiments to analyze the effect of steroid hormones on the enzyme XO, which he knew to be involved in gout pathology. In his 1963 study, Roussos proved two important points, the first being that the male hormones androsterone and testosterone stimulate and enhance the activity of XO. Roussos demonstrated that this hormonal stimulation of autogenous XO (the body's own XO), in the livers of some males, causes an end product of purine metabolism, uric acid, to be formed in excess and to spill over into the blood.   Too much uric acid can lead to gout.

The second key observation made by Roussos was that the female hormones, including estrogen and progesterone, inhibit XO activity. This minimizes uric acid formation and reduces the susceptibility of women to gout.

Clues such as these helped Oster build his thesis. To him it seemed that the effects hormones have on the activity of XO could be a reason for the difference in the rate of atherosclerosis between men and women prior to menopause.

The Elusive Causes

"When I began to theorize that somehow XO in food might be a dietary cause of injury to the arteries, there was naturally no ready information about this in the medical literature, " Oster explains.

"Indeed, although the symptoms and results of atherosclerosis were known, causes had not been positively identified."

Oster discovered that the debate over what promotes and what inhibits atherosclerosis was as convoluted as the information was unreliable. Interestingly, the situation has not changed much since the day he first started researching the subject.

Another theory closely linked with the hypothesis that cholesterol and saturated fats in the diet cause atherosclerosis is that of "risk factors."

The concept of "risk factors" is borrowed from insurance companies. It has become enormously popular in matters of the heart.

The list of such suspected factors is lengthy. In 1981, a leading medical journal listed 246 coronary risk factors neatly divided into two categories: primary and secondary.

The primary risk factors include: elevated serum cholesterol, high blood pressure, smoking and lack of exercise.

The more significant of the secondary risk factors are considered to be: diabetes, obesity, stress, heredity, abuse of alcohol, personality type, and gender. However, obesity, once close to the top of the list, is no longer considered a serious factor in the promotion of atherosclerosis. The same switch has been made about alcohol. Alcoholics have been found to have a relatively low incidence of atherosclerosis. Some researchers have pointed out that moderate intake of alcohol can actually raise levels of a beneficial type of cholesterol called high density lipoprotein, which allegedly slows down the arterial disease process. However, conclusive proof is still outstanding.

Despite the lavish expenditure of taxpayers' money by the various health foundations and governmental agencies, the medical establishment has not pinpointed what in the diet causes the initial injury to the arteries. For some curious reason one theory has become popular, the theory that fats and cholesterol in food will cause atherosclerosis.

All of the studies attempting to prove this theory lack any acceptable scientific base. Such studies extrapolate either from animal experimentation or from epidemiology, the statistical analysis of the incidence of disease in a population or a community, which depends heavily on causation by way of association. The results of animal experiments and the conclusions of epidemiology can rarely be verified scientifically in humans. This fact raises a very important philosophical issue: namely, *what responsibility does a medical body have to the public concerning statements and guidelines it issues when the information in them has not been proven in the court of science?*

Scientific arguments aside, Oster realized from personal experience that the dictum of "lower your serum cholesterol and avoid saturated fats to prevent cardiovascular disease" simply does not work.

Atherosclerosis can be induced in animals in all sorts of ways. When the arteries of research animals are deliberately scraped by catheters inserted into the blood vessels, the irritation starts the atherosclerotic process. This is termed mechanical injury. As part of the natural healing process cholesterol infiltrates the blood vessel wall.

People with high blood pressure, hypertension, may be sustaining mechanical injury to the arteries. The turbulent flow of blood may stress arterial walls and irritate the fragile endothelial lining, initiating a lesion with the same end result as an XO-induced lesion. High blood pressure per se is not known to produce atherosclerosis. If, however, there is an injury to the artery wall, high blood pressure becomes an added insult and is likely to aggravate the condition.

An imbalance in body chemistry may precipitate the onset of atherosclerosis. The research team of Gruberg and Raymond, at M.I.T. has accumulated interesting evidence that in some people a metabolic imbalance, characterized by a vitamin B_6 deficiency, may contribute to atherosclerosis. This is referred to as the homocysteine theory.

Van Buchem in Holland has shown that a decrease of lecithin in the bloodfats is found in those suffering from atherosclerosis. In one clinical study it was shown that those men with more than 36 percent lecithin in their bloodfats were clinically free of atherosclerosis while those with less than 34 percent bloodfat lecithin had symptoms of the disease.

Clues exist like sentinel signposts along the way. Frequently, there's an intriguing parallel to Oster's work. Some of the clues point to cell function and what causes changes in it. In the 1950s Biskind discussed the "rapidly rising incidence of cardiovascular disease and the association of atheromatosis with lipid metabolism...."

In 1982, the Nobel Prize in Physiology and Medicine was awarded to three biochemists, Bergstrom, Samuelsson, and Vane, for their discoveries concerning prostaglandins and related biologically active substances which derive from phospholipids, the substance related to plasmalogen.

The November 1982 edition of *Science* magazine explains that prostaglandins are "potent chemical transmitters of intercellular and intracellular signals that mediate a diversity of physiologic and pathologic functions." Some of these functions may include regulation of blood pressure, regulation of blood clotting and vasodilation as well as regulation of fat and cholesterol metabolism. Nutritional factors which may interfere with prostaglandin pathways may contribute to a variety of maladies, which may include atherosclerosis.

Dr. Burton Sobel, the current editor of *Circulation* the journal of the AHA, has proposed that derivatives of phospholipids (lysophospholipids), which are powerful detergents, are responsible for heart beat irregularities. This hypothesis is similar to that proposed by Oster and Ross in their paper published in 1975.

Perhaps these clues are more valid candidates for research than the so-called risk factors. Ross always asks, "Are there other dietary or infectious agents, like XO, which can also damage artery linings and which could lead to the same final state, viz., atherosclerosis?"

The Myth Of Cholesterol Dispelled

Before any new idea in science can be accepted, prevailing medical dogma must be displaced. Lying in Oster's path, like a large boulder obstructing passage, is the hyperlipidemia hypothesis, the pet theory of entrenched medical orthodoxy. The rather simplistic and near-sighted premise that too much cholesterol and saturated fat in the diet raises serum cholesterol triggering atherosclerosis has been formulated on considerable conjecture.

This prevailing concept has popular currency despite the fact that it has never been scientifically proved. Day after day, year after year, newspapers, magazines, radio, and television bombard the public with information on how it can avoid the hazards of these supposedly dangerous foods.

Madison Avenue Medicine

The printed word has considerable effect and is durable, but consider the impact of television on Americans, who tend to confuse their screen heroes with the roles they play.

Robert Young has been an effective spokesman for Sanka coffee because people identify him with his role as television's Doctor Marcus Welby. The actor's remarks about Sanka's soothing effects on the nerves have been widely accepted as coming from a physician.

Among 1982 and 1983 TV commercials were those that featured a prominent veteran of the theater, John Houseman. His role as autocratic teacher of law, Professor Charles W. Kingsfield, in the popular dramatic series, "The Paper Chase" has transformed him into an authority figure for American audiences.

In the commercials the actor stands in his best Professor Kingsfield classroom pose, asserting with considerable dramatic emphasis: "Puritan knows you're fighting high serum cholesterol – and Puritan wants you to win."

John Houseman is a brilliant director and an outstanding actor. But his qualifications for speaking authoritatively about high serum cholesterol are questionable. Puritan Oil and other manufacturers are not on safe ground either when they assure the consumers that it is important to fight high serum cholesterol. Apparently, the vegetable oil producers have been misled by the vast body of misinformation on the dangers of high serum cholesterol.

Puritan is not, of course, the only company suggesting that its vegetable oil is an effective agent in lowering serum cholesterol. Many of the vegetable oils for sale have been described by their manufacturers as being effective in reducing blood cholesterol. On the shelves in the supermarket, the bottles of Puritan sport a bright red tag urging the consumer to take action: "Ask Your Doctor About Making Puritan A Part Of Your Cholesterol-reducing Diet."

Vegetable oil commercials are brimming with

misleading information aimed at the gullible public. The general message doesn't change although there are several different commercials. One ends with two beguiling offers:

1. Telephone an 800 number to get a coupon for 20¢ off on Puritan Oil
2. Send for an American Heart Association (AHA) recipe booklet.

The general consumer commonly confuses the American Heart Association (AHA) with the main medical body, the American Medical Association, or AMA. Therefore, the advice for taking advantage of the AHA offer appears to much of the audience as if a medical organization such as the AMA agrees it is necessary to lower serum cholesterol. In reality the viewpoint of the AMA is quite different. The AMA has voiced its concern:

"The anti-fat, anti-cholesterol fad is not just foolish and futile.... It also carries some risk."

The free information provided the public is in magnificent conflict.

As Josh Billings, the Art Buchwald of the nineteenth century, so succinctly philosophized: "The trouble with most folks isn't so much their ignorance as knowing so many things that ain't so."

The mass media continues to churn out cautionary articles with obsessive regularity, warning the public to avoid dangerous saturated fat and cholesterol.

Physicians are confronted with similar misleading warnings. They are also inundated by books and articles in the professional journals about the risks of high serum cholesterol. The cholesterol controversy rages among specialists. For some physicians the conflict has become so confusing that they have withdrawn from the baffling fray.

From the National Research Council to the Superintendent of Documents to the Department of Health and Human Services, to countless other agencies, the American public is showered with pamphlets, diet books, and cautionary, conflicting advice. And, as educated as the public has become, people have never been more confused. What can be more confusing for the public than to hear John Houseman convincingly advocate cholesterol reduction and then, in another commercial, to have him praise the quality of the beef in McDonalds with what seems to be an egg for breakfast in the background.

At the prodding of certain interest groups, the government has been urged, most improperly, to issue dietary guidelines for all Americans. In a democratic society this function should probably remain the responsibility of mothers and not that of the government.

Assurances are continuously made that the information on which the advice is based stems from experts who know what they are talking about.

Do they?

For several decades now, Americans have been cautioned to avoid foods containing saturated fats and cholesterol to maintain sound cardiovascular health. Americans were also advised to use more polyunsaturated oils. In the U.S. alone, consumption of polyunsaturated margarines and oils has nearly tripled since the 1950s. An industry has grown up and now flourishes around this new dietary requirement.

Consumer Reports magazine analyzed the trend:

"The nation has become cholesterol conscious

and there's little doubt that Americans are consuming less animal fat and much more polyunsaturated fat than they did a generation ago." And ...what has been the result?

As one skeptical expert pointed out in 1973, "Certainly, if polyunsaturates really did work as claimed, with millions of people purposely eating so much of these particular fats, we should have a significant reduction in heart attacks."

Is this the case?

Apparently not.

* A 1964 report in the *American Journal of Clinical Nutrition* noted that the amount of heart disease has not decreased; rather, it has increased.

* In 1970, the National Heart and Lung Institute said that "heart disease has increased...."

* In 1973, Edward Pinckney, M.D. who is the author of five books on medicine for the lay person and more than 100 scientific articles and books for the medical profession insisted that "...all forms of heart disease have actually skyrocketed."

Despite such comments, some agencies, such as the National Center for Health Statistics (NCHS), started reporting in the mid-1970s that for the first time the United States was experiencing a slight but consistent decline in the total number of coronary heart disease deaths. According to the NCHS figures the coronary heart disease death rate in the United States peaked in 1967-1968 and has been declining since then.

If these statistics are, in fact, correct, they may more likely reflect the drop in total fluid, homogenized milk intake per person, which according to the Department of Agriculture's 1980 figure, was down about 15 percent from the 1960 figure. This decrease in homogenized milk consumption, due in part to fears of cholesterol, is tantamount to approximately 15 percent less biologically available XO in the diet of Americans.

Interestingly, according to the Department of Agriculture, the *total* consumption of cholesterol during the same period remained relatively constant. This suggests cholesterol cannot receive credit for any observable drop in coronary heart disease deaths.

One informed observer, who at the time happened to be the Assistant Secretary for Health in the Department of Health, Education, and Welfare, explained that the reductions have been most dramatic for infectious heart diseases, hypertension, and rheumatic heart disease.

Since no one ever claimed that a low-cholesterol diet would help in these three categories, this hardly seems to be meaningful in the great low-cholesterol diet debate.

The Assistant Secretary then added, that even for coronary heart disease, mortality rates that had been rising relentlessly for decades flattened out during the sixties and now are declining a bit. The bit, when defined by the Surgeon General in 1979, worked out to 2 percent per year.

Nevertheless, the media began to focus relentlessly on this as a possible trend. It wasn't long before promising headlines about the decline in heart disease became commonplace.

One story supportive of the misleading claims appeared in the *New York Times* in the spring of 1982: "Reduction Is Seen in Heart Disease." Upon closer inspection, the article reveals that the "decline" was observed in a program for reducing high blood pressure. This is certainly a valid area of concern, but it hardly begins to comprise the entire "heart disease" picture.

Not widely publicized is the fact that the advice to follow a low-saturated fat and low-cholesterol diet simply hasn't worked. Lives are not being saved because of the public's heightened awareness of saturated fat and cholesterol in the diet. A great body of hitherto unheralded research supports this point. It also reveals other facts that are disquieting in their implications.

First, increased intake of polyunsaturates may have created an assortment of new health problems: increased risk of cancer, as reported by an international team of researchers in *Lancet*, July 1971 as well as premature aging because of newly synthesized trans-fatty acids in certain polyunsaturated products such as margarine.

Second, when an individual consumes a polyunsaturate, such as corn oil, which does not contain cholesterol, it may help reduce the total dietary ingestion of cholesterol, but it does not necessarily lower serum cholesterol. This fact is documented in research findings presented to the American Institute of Nutrition as well as in a report to the U.S. Senate by the Agricultural Research Service.

These facts run counter to the bulk of information from devotees of the low-cholesterol diet, information which is misleading, at the least, and possibly dangerous in some of its applications.

The Source of the Misleading Information

Results of various medical studies are sent to newspapers and magazines. The media gives equal space to public relations releases and to scientific reports, frequently without discriminating between the two.

How can the media be faulted for accepting information from medical organizations? Why should the press find it any easier than the general public does when it comes to following the tortuous, contradictory developments in the controversy over diet?   Even medical specialists struggle to keep score of the accomplishments and the near-misses in the war on atherosclerosis.

Everyone is unwittingly misled by newspaper and magazine articles when they state that the research they are reporting on was "well designed," a phrase which is often used and which establishes a premise.

But is the research being publicized really well designed?

General Motors, in the 1960s, was advertising that its new rear-engine Corvair was a great new design in automobiles. It took Ralph Nader's book *Unsafe At Any Speed* to point out differently.   A study is only as good as its design.   The Corvair's suspension was faulty. Consequently, the car was never safe to drive.   Similarly, if the framework of a study is faulty, the results will always be questionable - or outright dangerous.

Many studies tying cholesterol with atherosclerosis are based on epidemiology. It is often surprising for the lay person to learn that information on death certificates is frequently of questionable accuracy. The interpretation of death due to cardiovascular disease varies from country to country. Thus, the statistics from which epidemiologists have drawn their deductions are often unreliable.

Disconcerting, is it not, to learn that all those dire warnings about cholesterol and fats in foods and all those sunny assurances that heart problems can be avoided by cutting such foods out of the diet are no more than broad inferences drawn from epidemiology, inferences that the government insists must be labeled "Not Proven"?

The MRFIT Fiasco

One of the most expensive studies on diet and

heart disease ever undertaken, a study which was a costly failure although one would never guess so from its press releases, was the Multiple Risk Factor Intervention Trial (MRFIT) project. It was financed by the National Heart, Lung, and Blood Institute. The study lasted for ten years and cost $115 million of scarce research funds. One primary purpose of the study was to establish the relative contribution supposed risk factors, such as high serum cholesterol, have towards coronary heart disease.

In 1972, when the study began, some 361,662 male volunteers, aged 35 to 57, were screened at twenty-two medical centers in the United States and Canada. Out of this large group of men, 12,866 were eventually selected for the study, nearly all of them white.

It is an interesting aside to ask the question why it was necessary to screen so many individuals before the final selection was made if America is indeed afflicted with "mass hyperlipidemia", the disease invented by advocates of the dietary fat and cholesterol-atherogenesis theory? The facts simply are not borne out that the population of the United States or any other nation suffers from "mass hyperlipidemia," a phrase coined and promulgated with grant support by Dr. Henry Blackburn.

The 12,866 volunteers were chosen because they supposedly had the "highest coronary heart disease risk...."

The designers of the study selected men who:

1. had high blood pressure;
2. had high serum cholesterol (according to the study's parameters);
3. had a history of smoking; "64 percent of the

smokers in the study each averaged 34 cigarettes a day."

Despite glowing progress reports during the 1970s by the researchers who designed the study, the final outcome of this lengthy, expensive experiment proved very little because the major premise on which the study was based was faulty. Not widely publicized is the fact that the 6,430 men in the special intervention group who were put on medication to lower high blood pressure "had a 66 percent higher mortality rate than expected."

The October 9, 1982, edition of the British medical magazine, *Lancet*, abandoned its customary British reserve by bluntly stating: "The results prove nothing."

Science magazine and the *New York Times* both termed the results "inconclusive."

The medical community is, understandably, reluctant to acknowledge that the MRFIT work contributed little to the understanding of what factors are responsible for heart and circulatory disease. The March 18, 1983, issue of the *Journal of the American Medical Association* contains several letters which are critical of the MRFIT program.

In one of the letters, Philip R. J. Burch, Ph.D., of the Department of Medical Physics of the University of Leeds in England expresses his hope that "the intense preoccupation with conventional risk factors will now diminish and that the search for the genuine precipitating agent(s) might commence."

Carl Seltzer, Ph.D., of Harvard University notes in another letter that the "reason for the striking failure of the trial lies in its erroneous basic assumption that reductions in CHD [coronary heart disease] mortality would result from reductions in the three so-called major risk factors: cigarette smoking, levels of BP [blood pressure], and

SP [serum cholesterol]."

Quoting an editorial from the *American Heart Journal* by Sir John McMichael, Dr. Seltzer adds, "An immense effort has been devoted to the reduction of cholesterol levels in the blood by diet and by drugs, and it must now be concluded that these efforts have had no detectable influence on the course and development of coronary heart disease." Dr. Seltzer concludes by reminding the reader that "the Food and Nutrition Board of the National Research Council found no evidence that a reduction of cholesterol in diets will help prevent heart disease."

In a hard-hitting letter contained in the same issue, Oster succinctly outlined why MRFIT produced inconclusive results. He explained that its methods were based on an "erroneously modified" formula, and also that MRFIT neglected to consider phospholipids, such as plasmalogen. Oster writes:

> The fatal flaw of the MRFIT program lies in its planning. The aim was to develop a broad, long-range plan for the study, control, and possible prevention of coronary heart disease. It should have been common knowledge that CHD is but *one part* of atherosclerosis symptomatology and should not be a surrogate for the entire problem.... The obvious failure in the high expectations of the MRFIT undertaking will perhaps lead to a rethinking of the problem, altered premises, and redirection of diet-heart research efforts into channels encompassing all division of fat metabolism, including the important phospholipids.

Jeffrey A. Cutler, M.D., of the MRFIT research group replied to Oster's letter and to those sent in by other critics of MRFIT in *JAMA*. Criticisms were brushed aside with phrases such as "little data," "one-sided literature review...." and "largely irrelevant."

These are the usual answers given by those who plan and run studies such as MRFIT. Meanwhile, triple bypass operations are on the increase. Innovative techniques for symptomatic treatment of heart disease continue to dazzle. Yet what is being done about the *causes* of atherosclerosis?

Until the fuel crisis and energy crunch of the 1970s, and the import of small cars, Detroit blandly ignored criticism that large cars were not the answer to all of our transportation needs. Another factor was the cost of retooling. Detroit just did not want to have to change its approach. That would have meant losing its current investment, spending on new methods, and admitting error. The name of the game is saving money and face.

Suspect the Statistics

One of the most puzzling aspects of work like MRFIT is why its results were so meager. Why were the results inconclusive when MRFIT took ten years and cost $115 million? Was this in fact a "well-designed" study? After all, the study's designers made sure their volunteers had all the major "risk factors" associated with heart disease.

How sensible was it to focus so sharply on apparent "risks?" For well over a decade, the findings of his own research have allowed Oster to query the design of work such as this.

Exasperated with the continuing lack of scientific results, Oster wrote the article titled "The Decline of Common Sense and the Ascent of Computerized Non-Sense in Medicine." It was published in *The Journal of Applied Nutrition* in the winter of 1975. In it, Oster made sure to include a comment by Cornfield and Mitchell from *The Archives of Environmental Health*: "We would be farther along in our knowledge of the effects achievable by intervention if we had relied less on statistical procedures of doubtful applicability and more on quality and quantity of observation."

Oster explains that "for the past two decades we have witnessed the sad spectacle of computer-wielding statisticians dictating changes in medical thinking and reactions to unsolved problems. These technologists have produced alleged probabilities (risk factors) which tend to result only in biological improbabilities."

"Is it wise," he concludes, "to base studies mainly on epidemiology?"

In a May 1981 article, "What Everyone Knows About Diet and Heart Disease May Not Be True" *Consumer Reports* notes: "The most provocative evidence linking diet to heart disease comes from epidemiology."

Often considered a twentieth-century science, epidemiology originated in seventeenth-century England.

In 1662 John Graunt, a London haberdasher, published his magnum opus, *Natural and Political Observations...Made Upon the Bills of Mortality*, and thereby established the field of epidemiology. Graunt brought to light a diversity of facts about human life and disease that had not previously been appreciated. He was the first to notice that the numbers of births and deaths of males exceeded those of females (by the ratio of 14 to 13); he noticed, too, that despite their greater mortality, men had less morbidity than women. Graunt quantified for the first time the high mortality in children, noting that one third died by the age of five.

The record-keeping in England offered both the means and the stimulus for monitoring statistics on death and illness.

Scientists after Graunt continued to analyze

"dry" mortality statistics and so formed the foundation for the epidemiology of the twentieth century.

But just how reliable is epidemiology's testimony?

Not very, according to a number of specialists, whose admonitions range from delicate reproofs to blunt outrage.

As an ex-President of the AHA, Thomas N. James, M.D., should be considered as one of its spokesmen. He is not diplomatic about his views of epidemiology, and he revealed his sincere convictions in his Presidential Address to the American Heart Association's 53rd Scientific Session in November 1980, "Sure Cures, Quick Fixes, and Easy Answers" in which he stated:

> Epidemiologists have long recognized and publicly deplored the soft nature of the clinical data obtained from masses of people, data which they then subject to increasingly complex and sophisticated mathematical analysis. But, no matter how marvelous such an analysis may be, there is no escaping the fact that the entire initial basis so often is less exact, less reproducible, and less reliable than any of us would wish.
>
> When we advise the public that they should eat less saturated fat and cholesterol, it is seldom made sufficiently clear that this advice is based on reasonable deduction rather than scientific proof, that such advice may or may not be helpful to everybody, or could even be harmful to some, or that dietary modifications with due consideration...may be of little avail.

Criticism comes equally from those in the field. Alvan R. Feinstein, Professor of Medicine and Epidemiology at Yale University School of Medicine, protested at a symposium in San Francisco in February 1981: "I know of no other scientific activity that's been so naive, so inappropriate, and so unscientific in its lack of attention to the basic data."

Years ago at a medical conference, Oster asked a leading epidemiologist if he considered high blood pressure to be a risk factor for heart attacks. When the scientist answered affirmatively, Oster then asked him to explain the fact that the incidence of heart attacks in Japan is low despite the well documented Japanese tendency toward high blood pressure.

Oster recalls that the epidemiologist was most disconcerted by the question but finally recovered his composure sufficiently to give him an answer smacking of instant analysis.

"The Japanese don't like to die and go to their ancestors with the stigma of a bad heart. So deaths from heart attacks are called deaths from stroke."

Not a remark to please Japanese physicians.

Built on Sand

"My questioning of studies such as MRFIT have to do with the obsession with the so-called 'risk factors'," Oster explains. "If smoking and elevated serum cholesterol have not been scientifically proved as causes of heart disease, why theorize that changing them would reduce the incidence of coronary heart disease?

"But beyond this fundamental question, one finds serious flaws when the MRFIT methods are examined."

MRFIT based its methods of calculating how risk factors could be reduced, largely, on the results of a previous study called the Framingham study because of its location.

The formula cited in the Framingham study held that a 10 percent reduction of the serum cholesterol (SC) level in the population of the United States would result in a 24.4 percent decrease in coronary heart disease (CHD) incidence; a 50 percent reduction in SC would result in a 84.2 percent reduction of CHD incidence.

The flaw in this reasoning is that risk is equated with incidence.

It would be more correct to read the figures as follows: people whose SC level is 10 percent lower than that of the average are 24 percent less likely to develop CHD.

Oster has made another interesting point rarely considered by scientists.

"I question the rationale in trying to lower serum cholesterol. What about the possible damage that might result from lowering serum cholesterol? The Framingham study did show that the group with the lower SC were more prone to cancer."

Despite the lack of significant results, the designers of the MRFIT study continue to rationalize their failure. Even though the study may have had "inconclusive results," they say it served a useful function even if it did nothing more than raise the red flag on treating mild hypertensives.

When Oster questions the quality of the MRFIT design, he is not merely displaying hindsight. He has voiced his doubts for many years. He raised similar queries about the Framingham study. He is not alone in doubting the efficiency and quality of such studies. Since these studies were conducted, many of his peers have also aired their protests.

In 1972, E. H. Ahrens, Jr., M.D., of Rockefeller University, wrote to the Inter-Society Commission for Heart Disease to tell them that he joined "Dr. Oster in condemning the easy but unjustified equating of Framingham risk data.... Simply because the Framingham data (and other similarly derived descriptive data) are all we have to use, does not justify the extrapolations so widely made as to the results expected if cholesterol levels in a given population are reduced."

The final paragraph of Dr. Ahren's letter is blunt.

"To the extent that large prestigious bodies (AHA, AMA, NRC, and ICHD) hand out manifestoes to the public that cannot be supported in fact, they delude the public and weaken their own credibility."

In Oster's article "The Decline of Common Sense and the Ascent of Computerized Non-Sense in Medicine" published in *The Journal of Applied Nutrition*, Winter, 1975, Oster's message is aimed at those who continue to delude the public:

> Science recognizes no manifestos; it aspires to the truth. Propaganda, on the other hand, is half truth and often wishful thinking. One of those propagandistic manifestos of partial truth is the chapter on 'Primary Prevention of the Atherosclerotic Diseases' contained in the Inter-Society Commission Report for Heart Disease Resources, published in 1970 and revised in 1972.
>
> The Inter-Society Commission is mainly a creation of the American Heart Association. Since its report is one of the most quoted documents in the field, it should be considered as a responsible attempt at the true gospel. Its content should be beyond reproach, its scientific basis should be unassailable, its various documentations should show all sides of a problem, its tables and statistical analyses should be firmly documented, and if and when edited this should be mentioned. Unfortunately, in every one of these criteria the report is sadly lacking. It is propaganda, a reservoir of half truth designed to impress the uninitiated.
>
> It is tendentious in frightening the American people with awe and fear inspiring

data on the death rate of atherosclerotic disease and related high morbidity and demeaning the sponsoring scientific medical societies involved in its shallowness and in its superficiality.

One of the fathers of modern experimental medicine, Claude Bernard, has stated, 'If the facts used as a basis for reasoning are ill established or erroneous, everything will crumble or be falsified.' This statement can well be applied to the Inter-Society Commission Report on Primary Prevention of the Atherosclerotic Diseases.

It is generally admitted that there is no conclusive experimental proof that lowering serum cholesterol in humans results in prevention of atherosclerotic diseases. After patients have already suffered a myocardial infarction, elevated serum cholesterol is not as powerful a risk factor as the occurrence of such new calamities as cardiac arrhythmias, heart enlargement, electrocardiographic abnomalties, or intermittent claudication.

Indeed, the Inter-Society Report states that no statistical significance was reached in these studies, and the results were not conclusive as to the preventive value of dietary changes. It is thus difficult to comprehend why any true scientist would lend his name to the manipulation of inconclusive data to make them meaningful.

Attention must also be given to the message contained in the first Annual Report of the National Heart and Lung Advisory Council (1974), which announced: "We do not know how to prevent atherosclerosis or how to diagnose and treat it early and...we tend to obscure our ignorance by making it seem that a problem has been solved. We must face up to our ignorance in many matters and recognize that an entirely different type of knowledge than we now have will be necessary to fully solve these problems."

How Human is a Rabbit?

In 1908, the Russian scientist A. Ignatowski published the first paper on inducing atherosclerosis in animals. Since then, there have been a number of experiments with animals...all aimed at proving atherosclerosis can be caused by particular diets.

Ignatowski force-fed rabbits an alien diet of meat, eggs, and milk. The rabbits developed atherosclerotic lesions in the aorta (the main artery carrying blood from the heart to the rest of the body). Ignatowski then drew his obvious conclusion:

> Animal protein in rabbits' diet causes atherosclerotic lesions in their aortas.

In 1913, two more Russian scientists, N. Anitschkow and S. Shalatow demonstrated that atherosclerotic lesions could be consistently obtained in rabbits by the feeding of pure cholesterol dissolved in sunflower seed oil.

From then on, members of the medical establishment started assuming that cholesterol in the diet causes atherosclerosis in humans. Even though man is not a vegetarian by design; even though man is not a rabbit. For the better part of the twentieth century, the medical establishment has been obsessed with a presumed connection between serum cholesterol and the development of arterial lesions.

Extrapolating the results of animal experiments to atherosclerosis in humans is an unreliable venture and represents a very dangerous leap in logical reasoning. In the words of Dr. E. Pinckney:

> As a matter of fact, the entire concept upon which the present cholesterol controversy is based is unique and totally opposed to all previously accepted scientific thinking. That

> is, the explanation now being offered by all
> those who do believe that excessive cholester-
> ol in the blood is deposited *on* the walls of
> arteries, runs counter to today's knowledge of
> classical pathology.
>
> ...briefly, those who condemn high levels of
> cholesterol in the blood believe that this cho-
> lesterol can deposit itself on the artery wall
> and then filter *through* that artery wall to
> form its plaque.

Pinckney goes on to say, "to justify the excessive cholesterol-in-the-blood answer to heart disease would require an entirely new approach to the
cause of almost all disease."

Not an insurmountable problem, but one which
hasn't been resolved.

Ignatowski was the first to prove that changing the food of animals could induce atherosclerosis. Ignatowski's actual conclusion that diet-
induced atherosclerotic lesions in the *aorta* of animals has been misconstrued to imply that humans
could have dietarily-induced atherosclerosis of the
aorta. Even if this is true, it is not as life-
threatening as atherosclerotic injury in smaller arteries, because the lumen of the aorta is much
larger than that of the coronary arteries.

An equal amount of atherosclerosis in the a-
orta and a coronary artery will have vastly different consequences. It can be compared to the difference between a garden hose and a fire hose. The
coronary "garden hose" affected by atherosclerosis
cannot handle the volume of blood, whereas the a-
orta "fire hose" affected by atherosclerosis can
still handle the necessary blood supply with relative impunity.

To return to the question of applying the results of animal experiments to humans, it is important to remember that the physiological responses
in humans and animals are different. The hormonal

balances of humans and animals are not the same. Finally, the metabolisms and diets of animals vary from one species to another. For example, it is perfectly normal for many animals such as the rat or the guinea pig, whose metabolisms are different than that of man, to have high levels of XO in their serum.

Herbivores such as rabbits show the greatest sensitivity to diets designed to create atherosclerosis. When other animals are used, the results are not as convincing. By the time the experiments have been repeated with carnivores, the results are far weaker, and the correlation between diet and atherosclerosis is statisically insignificant.

The short intestinal tract of the carnivore is designed primarily to digest meat. Scientists have tried feeding dogs as much meat as they can eat, all day every day, for long periods, but at first it was impossible to produce hypercholesterolemia in dogs. The scientists then started tinkering with the animals' bodies. By removing certain glands and feeding the dogs totally alien diets, they were able to create hypercholesterolemia. But, is a dog the same dog when certain glands have been removed?

Different mammalian species contain different amounts of naturally occurring XO in blood and in milk. Some animals such as rats and guinea pigs have tremendous amounts of naturally occurring XO in milk and in blood serum, while humans, sheep, and dogs have little or no XO. Compiling the findings of two independent research teams, Oster has compiled the data into a table. The unique distribution of XO in different mammalian species should suggest to researchers investigating the connection between XO and atherosclerosis that studies involving lab animals may have virtually no significance for the human condition unless animals are used which resemble man in having little or no naturally occurring xanthine oxidase in milk and in blood serum.

Table 4

Distribution of Xanthine Oxidase
Activity in Milk and Sera
Of Various Mammalian Species

Species	Milk ImU/ml	Serum mU/l
Rat	187.2	101
Guinea Pig	149.9	125
Cow	103.9	142
Rabbit	99.2	24
Donkey	80.6	29
Mouse	79.3	423
Horse	15.3	40
Goat	10.7	1
Sheep	9.9	0
Man	7.3	0
Man (colostrum)	20.6	0
Cat	7.9	0.6
Dog	3.3	44

Zikakis et al, *Instrumental Analysis of Food and Beverages: Recent Progress*, Academic Press, (1983)

al-Khalidi, U. A. S., Chaglassian, T. H., *Journal of Biochemistry*, 1965, 97:318-320

All of the differences between man and animals make it difficult to extend the results of animal experiments to the onset of atherosclerosis in humans. Countless experiments have been tried, but none have been able to prove that the mechanism by which atherosclerosis is produced in rabbits, or other animals, is the same in Homo sapiens.

Another factor rarely discussed or considered when animal experiments are evaluated is that, frequently, the animals' arteries are deliberately damaged, scraped with catheters, to *create* lesions.

As early as the 1900s, it was known that local injuries to the blood vessels of animals caused by mechanical abrasion or by scraping resulted in a damaging buildup of plaque and cholesterol within weeks, no matter what diet the animals received. In either a human or an animal this is the natural repair process in response to injury to the artery wall. Calcification is often a part of the body's healing process in response to tuberculosis or to other slow-acting infections. The approach of those who seek to lower serum cholesterol to counter heart disease is as simplistic as would be the attempt to heal TB by lowering serum calcium levels.

Human Guinea Pigs?

Do we know what happens if omnivores such as humans are given the same sort of experimental diet tried on different animals? No, such data is not available. Humans, unlike laboratory animals, are not supposed to be expendable. At this point in time any information on humans comes from unverifiable epidemiological data.

What individual would willingly have his arteries scraped with a catheter to establish whether atherosclerosis can be started in this way? Who would willingly be fed abnormally large quantities of, say, pure cholesterol, in an experiment? Few, if any, volunteers can be expected for such study.

Cost is yet another important consideration. For accurate results, thousands of people would have to be tested. One hundred and fifteen million dollars was expended for the MRFIT study. Estimates of possible expenses for tests, even simple ones like those performed in the MRFIT study, are colossal.

The only conclusion that may be drawn from Ignatowski's animal experiments is that something in a diet which is not the animals' normal one can promote atherosclerotic lesions in certain animals.

Special Interest Groups

In a desperate attempt to stem the rising tide of atherosclerosis, physicians throughout the country are forced to resort to one widely accepted and widely used approach: trying to lower the individual patient's serum cholesterol, either by diet or drugs or a combination of the two.

The manifold problem here is that the approach does not save lives.

It does not work.

It hasn't worked in the several decades that it has been in vogue.

Yet, it has enjoyed a certain kind of success, and that is *commercial success!*

"For certain segments of the food industry, the diet dogma is a real winner," writes George V. Mann, Sc.D., M.D., Professor of Medicine and Biochemistry at Tennessee's Vanderbilt University School of Medicine. "They sell products with health threats and promises based on this rather untenable hypothesis."

One clear and undebatable sign that the medical world has failed to find an effective preventive treatment to the problem is the rising incidence of the true last-ditch operation: the open heart coronary bypass operation that is being done in increasing numbers.

From 1975 to 1980, some 540,000 bypasses were performed in the United States. By 1982 the number had increased to 165,000 coronary bypasses per year.

But even the bypass operation has come under fire. Some physicians now call it "non-essential plumbing" and claim the same ends can be attained by judicious medication.

Diet, drugs, surgery or medication. How does the layman sort out the pros and cons of such treatment?

Do any of the methods offer legitimate hope for the victim of atherosclerosis?

Good advice on the subject is hard to come by, since chances are that not even the trusted family doctor knows any more about the subject than the party line on cholesterol that all physicians have been fed over the years.

Consumer Reports, the non-profit publication of the non-profit Consumers Union, hardly seems the place to go for medical enlightenment. Their stated purpose is "to provide consumers with information and counsel on consumer goods and services." Yet, *Consumer Reports* had its say on the subject of health and food in its May 1981 issue. In a feature entitled "What Everyone Knows About Diet and Heart Disease May Not Be True," *Consumer Reports* warned its readers that "There are widespread misunderstandings about the effect that diet can have on the incidence of heart disease."

The article pointed out that there is no acceptable evidence that cholesterol-rich, fat-rich diets have any meaningful effect on the level of serum cholesterol in the bloodstream. They revealed that diets artificially low in cholesterol and high in polyunsaturates posed health problems that are not really understood at present and could be harmful to growing children. All in all, this stalwart defender of the consumer public totally debunked the dietary programs that are often considered the answer to heart disease.

Yet, few people probably heeded the advice of such an article over that of a family doctor. An article in February 1982 *Fortune* magazine described Consumers Union as America's "most influential" organization of its type, yet very few are willing to accept its opinion in place of "good old Doc."

So, where *does* one go for advice?

Réné Dubos, in his introduction to *Anatomy of an Illness*, by Norman Cousins, reinforces the basic theme of the book and maintains that each individual, to some degree, must take charge of his or her own health before recovery from disease can be expected. "Every person must accept a certain measure of responsibility for his or her own recovery from disease or disability."

In his perennial bestseller, *Sugar Blues*, author William Dufty beseeches his readers to take responsibility for their own lives, to ask questions. The forsaking of this personal responsibility can only lead to the manipulation of a person by special interest groups which are often motivated by profit rather than humanitarian objectives.

People who have for any reason been advised by their physicians to change their serum cholesterol either by following a cholesterol-lowering diet or by using drugs (sometimes both), might well ask their doctors the following questions.

1   What is cholesterol?
2   Is serum cholesterol the same as cholesterol in your food?
3   How does changing the food I eat alter my serum cholesterol?
4   How do I know if my serum cholesterol is normal?
5   Are the drugs used to alter serum cholesterol safe?
6   Why is it necessary to lower serum cholesterol?

The Cholesterol Fallacy Exposed
Six Straight Answers

1. *What is cholesterol?*

A waxy alcohol, soluble in fat solvents (ether, petroleum ether, acetone or hot alcohol) but not in water, cholesterol is an integral part of the tissues of animals and people although it is completely absent in plants. Because it is a fat-like substance, cholesterol is often, wrongly, considered a fat.

The body manufactures cholesterol. Also, cholesterol is present in the food humans eat. Each day a normal adult synthesizes about 2,000 mg of cholesterol and eats anywhere from 300 to 600 mg.

A look at the role of cholesterol in the body reveals it is an indispensable part of cellular membrane structure. Medical scientist Michael S. Brown of the University of Texas Health Sciences Center explains: "Cholesterol is like a brick used to construct the wall between the inside and the outside of a cell."

The liver, which produces 1,000-1,500 mgs of cholesterol daily, is the body's main site of cholesterol synthesis. Small wonder, for the liver (the body's largest solid organ, usually weighing about four pounds) is an incomparable chemical plant. However, each person has numerous other sites at which substantial quantities of cholesterol are produced. These include the adrenal cortex, the intestines, the skin, the testes, and the aorta. Every tissue is capable of producing some cholesterol.

Over 90 percent of the cholesterol in the human body is found inside cells, where it participates in such essential functions as the formation of cell membranes and the production of sex hormones, corticosteroids, and bile acids.

Cholesterol that isn't used by the cells (a significant amount) or deposited on the walls of blood vessels (a miniscule amount) goes through another process; with the help of ascorbic acid it is converted by the liver into bile acids which help emulsify fats in digestion. Remaining cholesterol is either partly reabsorbed or excreted in the feces. Biochemicals are rarely reabsorbed unless they serve some useful purpose. For cholesterol to be carried in the bloodstream, it must be attached to receptors on water-soluble proteins, known as lipoproteins. Only since 1969 have the Framingham researchers recognized the long-known fact that cholesterol is transported in the blood plasma by lipoproteins. Cholesterol is distributed in the blood by four primary serum lipoproteins: high density lipoprotein (HDL), intermediate density lipoprotein (IDL), low density lipoprotein (LDL), and very low density lipoprotein (VLDL).

Cholesterol is also an effective insulator. It is primarily cholesterol that separates the individual electrochemical reactions taking place in each of the active brain and nerve cells. If such cholesterol were removed, a person's thoughts, mobility, indeed, a person's life would cease almost instantaneously because all the electrochemical processes, no longer shielded from each other, would immediately "short circuit."

The male and female hormones have as their precursor the cholesterol molecule. As a raw material cholesterol is especially needed by growing children.

Cholesterol is, in short, essential to life!

No one food is composed exclusively of cholesterol. Saturated fatty acids and cholesterol are found in abundance in fatty meats, eggs, butter and other dairy products, as well as certain shellfish like shrimp.

A diet designed to reduce intake of foods high in cholesterol and saturated fats would have to be very strict. For instance even skim milk contains cholesterol.

What happens when food which contains cholesterol is eaten?

Initially, cholesterol has to pass through the intestinal wall to enter the bloodstream. Because the intestine is limited in its capacity for absorbing dietary cholesterol, a normal adult could consume 600 mg of cholesterol in food in a day and only retain about 300 mg in the body, and of this amount, about 90 percent would be used by the body and the remainder eliminated.

The normal individual's body regulates the manufacture and absorption of cholesterol to suit its needs. In about 5 percent of the population, this mechanism goes astray, resulting in hypercholesterolemia. In such individuals the cholesterol "thermostats" fail for reasons poorly understood.

2. Is serum cholesterol the same as cholesterol in food?

Serum is the fluid part of the blood that remains after blood cells are removed by clotting. Cholesterol in serum is the same as cholesterol from any source, that which is created by the body or that which is obtained from foods.

3. How does changing the food I eat alter my serum cholesterol?

The answer to this question rips off the lid to a veritable Pandora's box.

First of all, when an individual is put on a diet to lower serum cholesterol, the impact on the person's life can be totally disconcerting. Such a diet tends to make every meal a tormented juggling of "okay" foods with the presumed-to-be harmful cholesterol and fat-laden foods. For most people a low-cholesterol diet takes away the pleasures of eating.

As an immediate consequence of a low-cholesterol diet, some people tend to become dietary hypochondriacs. Deciding what to eat and where to cheat causes inner tensions often not recognized by the dieter.

Oddly enough, inner tension is a critical concern because stress sends the level of serum cholesterol soaring. Increased cholesterol production is the body's reaction to tension much as the production of adrenalin is the body's reaction to a sudden stressful situation. As Pinckney explains, "the rise has no relationship to diet, let alone to the particular type of fat eaten."

"Soldiers have shown elevated cholesterol levels when they are required to perform any potentially dangerous mission."

An article published by John E. Peterson M.D. in 1960 noted that "blood cholesterol levels can vary by the hour." Dr. Peterson also demonstrated an even greater variation in cholesterol levels when subjects were exposed to various stresses, both physical and psychological. Psychological stress, however, seems to have the most marked influence on one's cholesterol levels.

In 1971, two U.S. Navy experiments indicated that cholesterol levels showed a profound rise whenever an individual was depressed or showed anger or fear.

A study presented to the 1971 meeting of the American Heart Association established "extremely sensitive" blood cholesterol levels resulted when medical students were subjected to "extreme stressful situations."

Even earlier in 1960, an article in the *American Journal of Medical Science* explained that cholesterol levels "more than doubled when a patient underwent any severe emotional stress."

Tension sends cholesterol pouring into the blood vessels. Any of life's daily aggravations can activate stress, a traffic jam or an unbalanced check book.

Table 5

SCATTERED VALUES OF SERUM CHOLESTEROL IN A GROUP OF INDIVIDUALS AT VARIOUS TIMES

Key:

○ = Low caloric diet, fasting   □ = High caloric diet, fasting
● = Low caloric diet, post-prandial   ■ = High caloric diet, post-prandial

Group A–G is male   **Group H–N is female**

Patient→ Serum Level ↓	A	B	C	D	E	F	G	H	I	J	K	L	M	N
150–159										■				
160–169		■												
170–179				●	□					□	□ ■			
180–189			□		○■ ●	□			●					□
190–199		○ ●	■	○				□ ■		○	○			■
200–209			●	■		■					●		□ ■	
210–219		□	○	□			■	○ ●						
220–244	■					□		○■ ●				○□ ■		
245–259	●							□				●		
260–284	○ □													

Note: Accuracy of determinations, by the Libermann-Burchardt method, was ≈3.5%.

Studies that date back to 1958 document an "acute rise in laboratory-measured serum cholesterol that occurred in tax accountants at the height of the tax season, in students during exam period, and in military personnel undergoing stress...with absolutely no change in diet."

Oster has demonstrated that "the same individual has variable values of serum cholesterol on different days, different seasons and other circumstances." In a paper published in *Medical Counterpoint*, April 1972, Oster included three tables on serum cholesterol levels. One of these, Table 5, is presented here. It points out how cholesterol values fluctuate within the same person before and after meals (post-prandial).

The co-enzymes (vitamins) and minerals required for the synthesis of hormone-like prostaglandins, which are believed to help regulate serum cholesterol, are depleted more rapidly during stress. This may be a significant factor in elevated, stress-related cholesterol increases. Oster noted many years ago, after examining one autopsy case, that sudden shock, which caused the collapse of the adrenal system, also caused plasmalogen depletion, the end-result being the same as that caused by XO.

Second, when cholesterol is eliminated from the diet there is rarely any meaningful effect on serum cholesterol. Strict vegetarians, for instance, who never eat meat, fish, or dairy products have serum cholesterol levels that almost match those of people whose diet includes all foods.

Third, if the amount of cholesterol in food is artificially reduced by diet control or with drugs, the body automatically manufactures more of its own. Dr. Myron E. Tract, Professor of Pathology at Columbia University College of Physicians and Surgeons compiled a list of commonly used drugs that will cause false results when blood cholesterol is measured. The report, which was published in 1972 showed that out of 49 drugs studied, 26 altered the cholesterol level sufficiently to yield an error in the test results.

Medical World News reported in the 1970s that the steroid drug cortisone causes the blood cholesterol level to rise significantly. Indeed, various hormones, whether produced naturally or taken as medicine, will severely alter one's blood cholesterol.

The body has "neurogenic control" over cholesterol production. Sensors regulate the *correct level for each individual* (with the rare exception of the hypercholesterolemic whose sensors function inefficiently).

One medical expert explains: "...if you do reduce the amount of cholesterol you eat, you are also signaling your body to manufacture more cholesterol on its own."

Fourth, as dedicated and as austere as a person may be about a low-cholesterol, high polyunsaturated diet, after about six months the body has a "tendency to start back up to its original cholesterol production level no matter how strict one is about the types of fats one eats."

Fifth, people who embark on the cholesterol-lowering adventure do not always experience anticipated results.

Pinckney explains: "Those on a cholesterol-lowering diet tend to develop more illnesses, including tumor, than those who eat a normal, well-balanced diet." Pinckney adds, "Worse, those who eat an excess of polyunsaturates seem to age prematurely and appear much older than they really are."

Patients advised by their physicians to follow such diets are not warned of these adverse reactions. Instead, they hear and read that countless studies have shown the *benefits* of lowering serum cholesterol.

The shortcomings of such studies are rarely cited nor are the comments from those who have voiced their concerns. Dr. Mann, the physician responsible for the evaluation of the dietary portion of the risk factor Framingham study, said that the entire concept of altering the kinds of fat one eats to reduce atherosclerosis is "overpromoted and overpublicized." Dr. Mann further elaborates: "We have not seen any evidence that these diets are effective." He uses words like "myth" and "wasteful diversion" to describe the cholesterol-lowering diet as something that lacks "convincing evidence in its support."

Convincing laboratory evidence which shows cholesterol in the diet has little to do with serum cholesterol levels has been brought to light by Goldstein, Kita, and Brown who explain in *The New England Journal of Medicine*, August 4, 1983, that separate pathways exist in rabbits for the transport of exogenous (dietary) and endogenous cholesterol.

4. *What serum cholesterol level should a person have?*

When the cholesterol level is defined to be 300, this indicates that for each 100 ml of blood, 300 mg of cholesterol are present.

The concept of labeling serum cholesterol as a harbinger of heart disease was initially developed in the 1950s. At that time a level greater than 150 was, in the estimate of the cogniscenti, "considered pathological."

Two decades later, there was a reassessment.

The "norm" of 150 established in 1950 was hastily discarded. A value of 300 became what was "in most cases considered within the range of normal."

The accepted standards seem to fluctuate according to the the whims of the health professionals.

In its 1974 handbook for physicians and dieticians, the National Heart, Blood and Lung Institute presents the following information.

Table 6
Table of Concentrations of Cholesterol which, if Exceeded, Clearly Indicate Hyperlipidemia

Age	Mg. per 100 ml.
1 - 19	230
20 - 29	240
30 - 39	270
40 - 49	310
50 -	330

In the 1980s, the medical community was pushing for a "norm" of under 200. Normal is a relative concept. The American Heart Association suggests that anything over 220 is abnormal.

If a physician suspects a person's serum cholesterol is higher than he believes healthy, a person might first ask whether it falls in the "norms" established by the National Heart, Blood, and Lung Institute, but even then many other factors must also be taken into consideration.

Serum cholesterol is one of the most highly variable factors measured in blood chemistry analysis. Each range for each individual is unique.

It appears the advice of many physicians for their patients to lower serum cholesterol as a precautionary measure against heart disease has no proven value.

Although physicians know that the results of most tests, such as those for hemoglobin, uric acid, and certain minerals are precise, they have found that the lab test to determine serum cholesterol level is not at all precise. This particular test is subject to more errors and variations than almost any other laboratory procedure.

This indicates that even highly skilled technicians can not be sure just how precise they are when reading the results of serum cholesterol level tests. It is extremely difficult to obtain an accurate reading.

Additionally, something often overlooked is the fact that some blood chemistry measurements, such as that of hemoglobin and of uric acid, do not change significantly as the years go by. It is crucial to take age into consideration when determining serum cholesterol. It is clearly documented that as one grows older, the serum cholesterol level increases.   This is neither bad nor good, merely a change that a physician and the lab technician, in particular, should always take into consideration. And, once again, it has never been scientifically proved that high serum cholesterol suggests problems!

Heritage is still another major influence on serum cholesterol.

Pinckney notes that "People of Southern European descent seem to have a much higher cholesterol level at all times in their lives than do those with an oriental background.   Those who have Scandinavian lineage would 'normally' be expected to have a higher cholesterol value without really indicating any abnormality of the heart."

It has already been explained that tension causes the flexible serum cholesterol level to fluctuate. Still other factors need to be considered, information that is generally kept from the public. People with Type A blood normally have significantly higher blood cholesterol levels than those with blood types such as B, AB, and O.

Certain conditions such as kidney disease, gallstones, hypothyroidism (low thyroid function), trouble with the pancreas, even pregnancy, can cause an individual's serum cholesterol level to go up significantly.

If a physician says that serum cholesterol is "elevated," or "too high" this does not automatically imply the individual has an excessive concentration of cholesterol and triglyceride (fats) in the blood.

Determining whether serum cholesterol is normal requires careful consideration of many factors.

5. *Are the drugs used to alter serum cholesterol safe?*

A great many drugs have side effects that are undesirable. However, this is yet another aspect of the "lower-your-serum-cholesterol-level" mania that has to be read to be believed.

As preposterous as it may sound, the law requires that "a drug to lower cholesterol cannot be advertised to the physicians without including a prominent statement to the effect that no one knows if the drug really works, whether lowering cholesterol will do any good whatsoever and that, in fact, the effect of the drug might be harmful."

The statement that the drugs "might be harmful" has corroborative evidence. Disastrous experiences have been recorded when drugs have been used to lower serum cholesterol. One leading exponent of the "lower-your-serum-cholesterol-avoid-heart-problems" litany, advocated that men take "large doses of estrogens to lower their cholesterol levels...."

The rationale was based on the fact that premenopausal women have less heart disease than men of the same age, probably because these women receive some measure of protection from estrogens. The effects of the female hormones on the men were difficult for the men to accept, the report noted. Most of the men were more prepared to face nausea, vomiting, and other stomach complaints than the enlarged breasts, loss of libido, and impotence caused by the female hormones.

A 1972 project used the cholesterol-lowering drug, dextrothyroxine (the commercial name is Choloxin) on patients who had a previous heart attack or coronary thrombosis. The FDA allowed the project to proceed, despite the drug's known side-effects and the warnings on the drug manufacturer's insert, provided with the drug; this explained it was inadvisable to use the drug on patients with a history of heart disease. If this had occurred in normal practice it might have been considered medical malpractice.

The researchers in the study maintained that it was double blind. This meant the patients and the researchers didn't know which patients were receiving a placebo or the medicine being tested. However, estrogen had obvious side effects, such as nausea, loss of facial hair, and breast enlargement. Clearly, when patients on the drug suffered these side effects, they and everyone else knew they were on the drug and not on placebo. The test was therefore neither secret nor double blind.

The research was undertaken in an attempt to protect against illness or death from heart problems. The project, a dismal failure, had to be ended prematurely. The group treated with the Choloxin had 18.4 percent more deaths than those in the parallel placebo group, despite the fact that the group on the drug had cholesterol values which were about 10 percent lower than levels generally considered "normal."

Two serum cholesterol lowering drugs, triparanol (commercially known as MER/29) and clofibrate (Atromid-S) possess known, extremely serious, side effects. Triparanol's side effects include

cataracts, baldness, and impotence. Even so, the
FDA cleared its use. Clofibrate, when used in major double blind studies, was reponsible for an increase in gallbladder inflammation serious enough
to cause gallstones and tumors which required surgery. Banned in other countries, Atromid-S is still
sold in America by Ayerst Laboratories. As a
clear-cut demonstration of the blind faith physicians have in drug advertising, clofibrate was once
the second most prescribed drug in the United
States.   Triparanol, however, is no longer on the
market.   Close to $20 million in damages were
awarded to victims of its side effects because the
manufacturer had withheld pertinent information
about the known side effects.

How should one feel about taking drugs with
known side effects? If a drug were known to be
lifesaving a person might, after weighing the pros
and cons, decide to tolerate a drug's known side
effects to rid himself of some dread disease. In
the case of the cholesterol-lowering drugs, the
risks far outweigh potential benefits. This is crucial information which seems to have been deliberately ignored and obscured by people with a stake
in promoting the "lower-your-serum-cholesterol"
myth.

In the *Journal of the International Academy of
Preventive Medicine*, published in 1983, Oster rei-
terates: "The doubt about the search for an optimum serum cholesterol was also expressed recently
in an article appearing in *Lancet* (Kannel and Gordon, 1982) where it is stated: 'We must admit to a
certain *regret* (sic) that there does seem to be a
gradient of CHD risk at low levels of serum cholesterol.' The basic policy fault, in my opinion,"
Oster adds, "is that the AHA reports equate CHD
with atherosclerosis."

The rather scandalous truth is that time and

millions of tax dollars have been spent on choles-
terol research. Dr. Mann explained in the 1970s
that the "myth...has been a terribly wasteful diver-
sion for the medical community.   After twenty
years and several hundred million dollars, we still
do not see any convincing evidence in its support."

So much time and effort – yet no proof exists
to date that lowering cholesterol makes any differ-
ence to people who suffer from atherosclerosis,
whether they have coronary heart disease or other
vascular disease. The bitter irony is that the medical establishment's most widely used preventive
approach to atherosclerosis appears to be a cruel
sham.

6. *Why is it necessary to lower serum cholesterol?*
    The answers to the previous five questions in-
dicate that no verifiable proof exists that lowering
serum cholesterol does any good for anyone.

    Does the medical establishment have some
reason for their monumental concern over the dangers of cholesterol? Not really and, unfortunately,
as Pinckney has noted, "when the American Heart
Association, margarine manufacturers, and certain
governmental health divisions tell the American
people that cholesterol is bad, the physician who
questions this edict, asking for some sort of proof,
is considered out-of-step."

    However, those in the medical establishment
who insist that cholesterol is dangerous say that
their hypothesis has been proven because cholesterol comprises part of the atherosclerotic plaques
that clog arteries.

    How true is this?

    Association does not imply causation.

    Whether serum cholesterol is high or low, if
the arterial lining has been damaged by an irritant

(whether a viral or bacterial infection or XO or some other toxic substance) an atheromatous plaque, the raised patch or buildup of deposits, usually yellowish in color, found on the inner surface of an artery.

It is in this second stage, when there is the buildup of deposits, that cholesterol is found, in the form of a chemical compound referred to as an ester. Cholesterol is an alcohol, a fatty acid is an acid. When an acid is mixed with an alcohol, a compound known as an ester is produced.

Once again, cholesterol is *not* present in the first stage of atherosclerotic development. First comes the damage to the arterial lining, *then* the buildup.

Despite years of experiments at a cost of billions, no scientist has ever been able to prove that cholesterol causes that initial damage in humans. The claim that cholesterol is the initial cause of the atherosclerotic plaque is not based on fact.

The results of lowering serum cholesterol with drugs is not a reasonable alternative, for the results may be downright dangerous.

The actual scientific facts on lowering serum cholesterol add up to something quite different from the accepted "wisdom" that has for so many years been preached by the advocates of diets to lower your serum cholesterol.

Kurt Oster's revelations consistently fly in the face of the testimony arrayed by the animal experimenters and the epidemiologists. Thus, he has come under bitter attack from that part of the medical establishment whose ideas have long since been formed and set in concrete. Oster and Ross are now working at presenting their evidence to a younger generation who have noticed the chipped plaster in the old edifices.

Politics

The Federal Trade Commission
vs.
The National Commission on Egg Nutrition

It is spring 1975, in the city where the business is government; Washington, D.C., the legislative, administrative, and judicial center of the United States.

One of the government agencies, the Federal Trade Commission (FTC) is suing the National Commission on Egg Nutrition (NCEN), accusing them of false and misleading advertising.

"You must prove your statement that 'no scientific proof exists that eating eggs causes heart attacks'," the FTC had told the NCEN.

Oster was there because he had agreed to testify for the NCEN, the defendant.

"Good morning, sir," the usher opened the door of Room 7312 and nodded to the man who came hurrying along the corridor of Building 1101.

"Good morning. Ah, I'm not the last one."

Oster paused for a moment and looked around the room.

The three attorneys representing the FTC, a woman and two men, were clustered on the right-hand side of the room conferring in low voices.

At the sound of footsteps, he turned and saw the attorneys for the NCEN, heads together in earnest conversation as they strode briskly along. The senior man looked up and smiled when he caught sight of Oster.

"Morning, doctor. Good to see you."

Oster returned the smile. He knew the NCEN was glad to have him in Washington to testify in their behalf. Apparently he was the only physician in America with accepted research credentials willing to accept the NCEN's invitation.

"Just about everyone else we've called so far has declined. They say their schedules are too heavy," the spokesman for the NCEN explained when he approached Oster.

"Do you know who will be testifying for the FTC?" Oster asked curiously.

"I believe Doctors Stamler, Connor and Blackburn, among others."

"Of course."

Oster would have been astonished if those names had not been listed. They were the heavy hitters of the cholesterol controversy, the Babe Ruth, the Hank Aaron, and the Reggie Jackson of the Ban the Egg Team.

The dictum "lower serum cholesterol and avoid heart problems" has a mammoth following in the United States. The debate over cholesterol and saturated fats in the diet has continued for decades.

Also pouring in for decades has been the financial assistance for studies that have sought scientific proof to support the claim. The proof is still missing.

"We do have two British specialists who're willing to testify for us," the NCEN spokesman explained.

Oster was almost certain he could predict who these two were.

"Doctor Oliver, University of Edinburgh and Doctor Yudkin, University of London."

Exactly as Oster had thought. For years, these two distinguished scientists had spoken out with the vocal minority. Both have insistently pointed out that no scientific proof exists that lowering cholesterol "will do any good whatsoever."

Oster's attention was brought back to Room 7312. The judge had entered. Within minutes the proceedings had picked up from the point of the previous day's adjournment.

The hearings had already lasted for weeks.

Oster was thankful his presence was needed for only one day. The preparation with the NCEN legal counsel beforehand had been incredibly time-consuming. During the day he had to be in Washington, he spent the entire time in Room 7312, where he was called to the stand. He listened with great interest to the attorneys' questions and the replies.

He resolved to read the transcript when finally the case was over. That resolution shrivelled and died when he found the typewritten pages numbered close to a thousand.

That spring the American public had other news vying for their attention. The United States was in the grips of a severe economic recession. Unemployment figures were high. Haldeman and Erlichman were sentenced to prison for their role in Watergate. Then, in the aftermath of bloody coups, as Communist forces overthrew the pro-American governments of South Vietnam, Cambodia, and Laos, some 150,000 Vietnamese refugees fled to the United States. When Cambodia seized the U.S. merchant vessel *Mayaguez*, U.S. Marines attacked and rescued the hijacked ship while the world watched.

Provocative Ads

The legal proceedings that took place in Washington early in 1975 probably could not compete for the public's attention. Indeed, Americans might not even have been aware that the FTC, in its desire to ensure "truth in advertising" and live up to its role of "guardian of the people," deemed it necessary to sue the NCEN.

From June 31, 1980, to June 30, 1981, the U.S. Government prosecuted some 32,000 lawsuits, and the FTC's share of these was considerable. This was reason enough for the casual reader to lose track of issues.

Whatever the public did or did not read about the suit, they could hardly have missed the series of advertisements placed by the NCEN in newspapers around the country that had prompted the lawsuit; the first that Oster noticed appeared in the *Washington Post* in January 1975. Its tone was strong and sober, the headline bold: *"A British Study Has Found No Evidence That Eating Eggs Is Related to a Risk of a Heart Attack."*

Two of the advertisements are shown on the following pages.

A Critique of Credentials

When at last Oster was on the stand, one of the attorneys for the FTC made a surprising request. It was so unusual that not even the possibility of it had been mentioned to Oster in the briefings by the NCEN counsel before the hearings.

The FTC attorney asked the judge to disqualify Oster. The request was based on the fact the Kurt A. Oster, M.D., was a practicing physician,

A BRITISH STUDY HAS FOUND NO EVIDENCE THAT EATING EGGS IS RELATED TO A RISK OF HEART ATTACK:

Cholesterol

"In certain animal species a diet rich in cholesterol induces the appearance of arterial lesions which have some similarity to those seen in human subjects, and comparative studies of different human populations show that those which have a diet rich in cholesterol have a higher death rate from I.H.D. However, a diet rich in cholesterol is usually one which is rich also in saturated fatty acids. Most of the dietary cholesterol in western communities is derived from eggs. **but we have found no evidence which relates the numbers of eggs consumed to a risk of I.H.D.**" * (emphasis ours)

> — *DIET AND CORONARY HEART DISEASE, a Report of the Advisory Panel of the Committee on Medical Aspects of Food Policy (Nutrition) on Diet in relation to Cardiovascular and Cerebrovascular Disease. Issued by Britain's Department of Health and Social Security.* An official British Government report, published in London in 1974, by a panel of Great Britain's most distinguished physicians, researchers and nutritionists.

The American public too has the right to this information.

NATIONAL COMMISSION ON EGG NUTRITION
Park Ridge, Ill. 60068

* Ischaemic Heart Disease (coronary heart disease) is a cardiac disability (either acute or chronic) which arises from a reduction or an arrest of the blood supply to part of the heart muscle either by a narrowing of a blood vessel or by complete obstruction of it.

THE NATIONAL COMMISSION ON EGG NUTRITION BELIEVES THE AMERICAN PEOPLE SHOULD HAVE THESE FACTS

Hundreds of millions of dollars, much of it government money, have been spent on research projects attempting to prove that lowering blood cholesterol through diet or drugs will reduce the risk of heart disease. The search has proven fruitless.

Here are three studies reported in 1975 which help clarify the question as to whether or not eliminating eggs from the diet will lessen the risk of heart disease.

1. At UCLA, Dr. Roslyn Alfin-Slater, and others. selected two groups of healthy, male subjects who normally ate eggs and whose serum cholesterol and blood pressure were in normal range. One group, 25 men whose age ranged from 20 to 28 years. were fed two eggs per day for eight weeks in addition to their usual cholesterol-containing diet. The other group, 27 men with an age range of 39 to 66 years, were fed one egg per day for four weeks. then two eggs every other day for four weeks. For two weeks after the eight-week feeding period. all eggs were removed from that diet. Serum cholesterol determinations were conducted on two successive weeks before the egg diets were given, weekly for eight weeks during the egg feeding, and thereafter on the egg-free diet. The results indicate that there were no significant differences in average serum cholesterol levels between any two time periods in either group. (Reported at the International Congress of Nutrition. Kyoto. Japan, August 8. 1975.)

2. In a Minnesota study, half of a group of 17,000 patients in state hospitals — where diets can be strictly controlled — ate a normal diet and the other half a diet lower in cholesterol. After 4½ years, researchers totaled the number of heart attacks, strokes, and other cardiovascular problems that affected people in each group. Dr. Ivan Frantz. of the University of Minnesota, who reported on the projects. stated: "In the entire population . . including men and women of all ages over 21, despite a satisfactory decrease in blood cholesterol. there was not the slightest hint of benefit." (Reported at the American Heart Association's annual Scientific Sessions. Anaheim, California, November 17, 1975.)

3. Dr. William Weidman. a Mayo Clinic researcher. reported on a three-year study which involved more than 2,500 school children. from six to 16 years of age. Dr. Weidman stated: "There was no correlation between the level of cholesterol in the blood and the amount of cholesterol in the food they ate." This study was financed by a $2.1 million grant from the National Heart and Lung Institute. a Federal agency. (Reported at the American Heart Association's annual Scientific Sessions. Anaheim, California. November 18. 1975.)

FOR YOUR ADDITIONAL INFORMATION . . .

The Coronary Drug Project was started in 1966. It was funded by the National Heart and Lung Institute at a cost of $40 million. The purpose was to determine whether lowering blood cholesterol concentration through use of drugs could prevent heart disease. At the start. 8,300 men were involved, upon which five drugs were to be tested. Three of the drugs were discontinued early in the tests because of undesirable side effects. The other two drugs. clofibrate and niacin were administered to the end of the test. The controls received a placebo (a "blank" capsule or pill which has no effect). Clofibrate and niacin are the most widely used cholesterol-lowering drugs. The serum cholesterol of those receiving the drugs was lowered more than is usually accomplished through stringent diets. At the end of the eight-year project, neither group receiving the drugs had a significantly different rate of heart disease than the group receiving the placebo. (Reported in the January 27. 1975. issue of the *Journal of the American Medical Association.*)

not a statistician. Therefore, the attorney reasoned, his credentials were not acceptable in this situation.

The judge gravely considered the attorney's request but did not permit the disqualification.

Although her opening gambit had failed, the FTC attorney maintained tight control of the situation.

The questions she put to Oster were brief.

The attorney knew Oster's position.

She knew Oster believed the advertisements run by the National Commission on Egg Nutrition were for the most part accurate.

She knew Oster believed eggs were a good, nutritious food which could be eaten without dire consequences.

Years later, Oster described the curious incident that happened after the day's proceedings were adjourned.

"I was about to leave the room, when the attorney for the FTC came up to me. 'Hope you didn't mind the treatment,' she said. 'Nothing personal. Just one of those legal maneuvers'.

"The point is, legal counsel for the FTC just plainly didn't want my evidence on the record.

"The questions I was asked by them were mostly about statistics. A lot of emphasis was put on the fact that I am not a certified biostatistician. Never mind that the other witnesses, those *for* the FTC, were not practicing physicians.

"Do *they* see patients day in, day out, year in, year out? My patients do have to eat, after all. My research work actually has involved studying patients under controlled situations, feeding them eggs in their daily meals, monitoring their serum cholesterol levels.

"Clearly, my knowledge and information about the effect of eggs in our diet and the effect of eggs on individuals with atherosclerotic problems is current. Cardiology is my specialty. I concentrate my medical research on the causes of atherosclerosis. In my medical practice, many patients come to me suffering from the symptoms of atherosclerosis. Can anyone legitimately deny my credentials in this field?

"I did my best. I explained that no scientific proof exists to relate the number of eggs consumed to a risk of ischemic heart disease. I told them I agreed to a large extent with what the NCEN ads said."

"The result was almost to be expected: The FTC had more witnesses than we did. More of their testimony was admitted. The opposition's testimony was accepted as accurate. Ours was not.

"Of course, by the time of the hearing, the spring of 1975, I had done far more for the NCEN than testify in the FTC lawsuit. I had agreed early in the year to go on tour, speaking on behalf of the NCEN. I travelled to many different places across the country. I made many public appearances for the NCEN. Television shows, radio shows, press conferences. They kept me very busy. My topic was of great interest to audiences everywhere."

Indeed, a public that had repeatedly been told of the dangers of too many eggs in their diet was fascinated to learn that their British cousins, and some of their resident medical specialists, held a different view.

"I told audiences everywhere that eggs are good food, that there isn't any proof to connect them with heart problems. I told them I believe in the information in the NCEN ads.

"Surely, time will prove eggs are a good food!"

Closing the Information Gap

In Washington, after listening to weeks of presentation and cross-examination, the FTC issued a ruling. It was the opinion of the Federal Trade Commission that the National Commission on Egg Nutrition had not proved their statements about eggs in their current advertising.

The NCEN was ordered to take all such advertisements off the market.

The was a remarkable example of one arm of the government not knowing – or believing, or caring – what another arm of the government says and does.

The United States government insists that "a drug to lower cholesterol cannot be advertised to physicians without including a prominent statement to the effect that no one knows if the drug really works, *whether lowering cholesterol will do any good whatsoever....*"

One claim is made by those who advocate reducing the quantity of eggs the public consumes. They claim that lowering serum cholesterol is helpful for those with cardiovascular problems, even though no scientifically verifiable proof exists to support that claim. Yet when a counterclaim is advertised another government branch, the FTC, forbids dissemination of the claim.

Rarely is the public presented with the type of information the NCEN put in their advertisements, information that, while closely accurate, runs counter to prevailing opinion.

Eggs Do Not Raise Serum Cholesterol

Political pressures frequently lead to distortions in the way medical research is reported – a fudging of issues.

Oster has been tireless in analyzing and exposing this kind of shoddy work. He can tread his way through the tangled undergrowth of the medical and biochemical research jungles. He can spot a weasel word at thirty yards and a slanted opinion at a hundred.

Included in the appendix of this book is the complete text of a letter he wrote, "The Egg Controversy: Are Eggs Good or Bad?" The letter, which deals with the issue of "fudging" was addressed to the editor of the *American Journal of Clinical Nutrition* and was published in the December 1982 issue.

As the letter's title suggests, this is a subject of almost universal interest. Most everyone eats eggs. Nearly everyone has heard the advice that it is supposedly wise to restrict consumption of eggs. As a consequence of such warnings, many people *do* avoid eating eggs daily. Some, it appears, even feel guilty about eating an egg every other day.

Oster has insisted over the years that eggs are one of the most nutritious foods available in nature. He contends strenuously that it is wrong to deprive people of this good, inexpensive, and easily obtainable food on theoretical grounds for which no iota of scientifically verifiable evidence exists.

Growing children need eggs. People on tight budgets can eat well because of them. The elderly, for whom simple, easy-to-prepare meals can make the difference between self-sufficiency and requiring outside help, should not be denied the convenience or the high nutritional value of eggs. An egg is a balanced food. It contains all of the vitamins that are found in a good multivitamin pill; it is simply one of nature's better foods.

In "The Egg Controversy: Are Eggs Good or Bad?" Oster discusses a study published in the

American Journal of Clinical Nutrition, October 1981. This study, "Does Egg Feeding (i.e. dietary cholesterol) Affect Plasma Cholesterol Levels In Humans? The Results Of a Double Blind Study," by S. L. Roberts, M. P. McMurry and W. E. Connor, makes a number of statements which are, as Oster carefully details, extremely misleading.

Some of the information in the title itself is not strictly accurate. The words "Egg Feeding," suggest the study used regular eggs. This was not the case. Careful perusal of the text reveals that the eggs used in the study were homogenized. An egg bought in a store anywhere in the world, however, will not be homogenized. In itself, homogenization of the product raises an important point, as Oster notes in his article:

> Just as homogenization of milk will produce increased bioavailability of an enzyme, xanthine oxidase [7], so will homogenization of an egg increase the biological availability of cholesterol. This was beautifully proven by Thompson et al [8] .... Connor ignores this biological fact and equates homogenized artifacts with the natural product of a shell egg.
>
> Another discrepancy can be found within the title of the Roberts et al, egg feeding study. The study was not actually "Double Blind." As Oster explains, the study was really a triple blind experiment. It depended on the manufacturer of the frozen homogenized whole eggs for the quality of the eggs.
>
> This in turn leads to an interesting consideration. The frozen homogenized whole eggs were prepared by Standard Brands, Inc., a commercial firm with a financial interest in promoting their product, Egg Beaters. Vested interests raise questions about objectivity.
>
> The authors come to the conclusion that feeding of whole eggs in a double blind study, to outpatients eating their customary diets, had a hypercholesterolemic effect compared

to a cholesterol-free product. They implied that the hypercholesterolemic effect contributes to an increase of atherosclerosis and heart attacks. They also stated that results of early metabolic experiments are confirmed. This research already has been incorporated as a key reference on diet. One does not doubt that the data presented are factual, but what is very much in question is the relatedness of the present study to other investigations [2-5] which have not found any significant changes in serum cholesterol with the addition of eggs to the home diet of adult men and women.

Also, the addition of two whole eggs to the regular diet of hospitalized patients have not shown any significant increase in serum cholesterol. My own unpublished studies of two hospitalized patients with a daily feeding of two eggs, extending over a period of two years, did not produce any serum cholesterol increase whatsoever. There was a minimal increase of 5 percent after the first month which returned to the original level and remained unchanged over the entire period of two years.

One wonders how such variance in results of egg consumption and cholesterol changes could happen, expecially since this issue was in the foreground of the Federal Trade Commission trial of the United States government against the National Commission on Egg Nutrition in 1975, in which Connor was a government witness. This discrepancy in scientific reports of finding no changes in serum cholesterol after shell egg consumption on one hand and elevation of serum cholesterol after homogenized egg consumption, on the other hand, needs definite scrutinizing analysis because so much has depended on the wording and the semantics applied in the claims and counterclaims.

A Vital Contradiction

The points that Oster raises in his article on

eggs are critical in understanding that "shell" eggs, which are regular, natural eggs unprocessed by the hand of man, do not raise serum cholesterol and in understanding why the results of Conner's work are invalid. The Connor study, in which homogenized eggs were used instead of "shell" eggs to demonstrate increases in serum cholesterol, is already part of the standard references on diet. It contradicts other standard works. Oster cites references 2-5 which showed consumption of cholesterol and eggs does not raise serum cholesterol. These works are included below, should the reader want to refer to them.

Reference number 2, a study by G. Slater et al, "Plasma Cholesterol And Triglyceride In Men With Added Eggs In The Diet," appeared in *Nutrition Reports International* in 1976. The following articles appeared in the *American Journal of Clinical Nutrition*: M. W. Porter, et al, published "Effect Of Dietary Egg On Human Serum Cholesterol And Triglyceride Of Human Males," in 1977; M. A. Flynn, et al, published "Effect of dietary egg on human serum cholesterol and triglycerides" in 1979; F. A. Kummerow, et al, published "The Influence of Egg Consumption on the Serum Cholesterol Levels in Human Subjects," in 1977.

These reports were unanimous in stating there was absolutely no case to be made against eggs; eating them will not cause a normal person to have a significant increase in serum cholesterol. There is no subsequent increased risk of atherosclerotic or cardiovascular problems.

The immediate effect of the 1981 study by Roberts, et al, is to contradict and question the studies mentioned above yet; the fact is, these were well-designed studies. It is the Connor study, as pointed out, which has questionable results.

In his letter, Oster raises another consideration. It is the same consideration that applies to his work on how homogenization of milk makes xanthine oxidase in milk "biologically available."

"I think there exists an urgent need for nutrition science to follow the example of pharmacology and pharmaceutical product preparation, both of which stress the importance of biological availability of a product. Disregarding this concept leads to unexplainable and nonscientific results causing unnecessary controversy. The concept of availability of a chemical is of utmost importance in generic drug research and should be grafted as a branch of scientific nutrition."

Oster is intrigued that so few researchers in nutrition understand how the homogenization of a food changes its properties. The concept of bioavailibility applies to any food, whether it is homogenized milk, or eggs, or anything else.

The article "Dietary Dogma Disproved," published in the April 29, 1983, issue of *Science*, contains revolutionary information on nutrition. It agrees with Oster's long-held view that the homogenization of a food makes it easier for it to pass from the gut into the bloodstream. The article explains that "the more homogenized the food, the more rapid the rise in blood glucose. A rice slurry gives a more rapid rise than rice grains. Apple puree gives a more rapid rise than a whole apple." The same researchers exploded the commonly accepted principle, taught to students in fundamental biology, that simple carbohydrates (sugars) such as glucose are taken up more rapidly from the gut. This produces a more rapid rise in blood sugar than complex sugars such as starch from potatoes.

One of the primary researchers in this area, Phyllis Crapo, of the University of Colorado Health Sciences Center in Denver recently made several key points:

1. Frequently prevailing nutritional dogmas are based on unproven assumptions and are often wrong.

2. The professional nutritionists believe such dogma even though *they have not been tested.*

3. What happens when food is eaten is much more complex than previously suspected.

4. The wholesale change in industrialized societies from foods like pasta, beans, and sweet potatoes to foods like bread, cereals, and white potatoes might be related to the prevalence of diabetes, *heart disease*, and some forms of cancer." (emphasis added)

Oster's background in pharmacology gives him an advantage over many specialists and researchers in understanding "biological availability." As important as this concept is to applied nutrition, few have considered it.

Oster points out in the last paragraph of his letter on homogenization of eggs:

> I suggest that Connor's equating homogenized eggs with shell eggs is unwarranted and scientifically untenable. It has been adequately shown by respected scientists [2-5] that eating shell eggs in a nonhomogenized form by normal persons will not cause a significant increase in serum cholesterol and therefore constitutes no subsequent greater risk of atherosclerosis and heart disease. It should be reasonably concluded that those who have no cholesterol metabolism problem may continue to eat shell eggs without putting their health in jeopardy.

The Elephant Who Delivered a Mouse

Specialists besides Oster are concerned about the care of people with atherosclerosis. If patients are advised to eliminate risk factors, is this enough?

The risk factor concept has aroused a great deal of controversy. Perhaps it takes someone who lives and works in another country, outside the boundaries of the political cloud hovering over physicians in the United States, to write an unusually blunt article for the *Journal of the American College of Cardiology*.

"Contribution Of The Risk Factor Concept To Patient Care In Coronary Heart Disease," by Frits L. Meijler, M.D., F.A.C.C., of the Netherlands, appeared in January 1983. Dr. Meijler is that *rara avis*, a non-American member of the American College of Cardiology. His article has a refreshing candor.

The Dutch cardiologist writes:

> This article deals with the question of whether or not the risk factor concept, a principal aspect of preventive cardiology, has contributed to patient care in coronary heart disease. The risk factors considered are plasma cholesterol, high blood pressure, smoking, diabetes and marked obesity. With the exception of plasma cholesterol and diabetes, all of these factors enhance myocardial consumption and thus, in the presence of coronary insufficiency, promote myocardial ischemia. Their modification is, therefore, good general medical practice, even if not related to coronary atherosclerosis....
>
> It has never been and probably never will be demonstrated that lowering plasma cholesterol levels by diet or other means will cause regression of coronary atherosclerosis. It follows that modification or treatment of risk factors is implemented for good medical reasons but does not *demonstrably* or *predictably*

affect coronary artery disease. It is concluded
that the contribution of the risk factor concept to patient care in coronary heart disease
has been, and still is, trivial.
   *The pillars of preventive cardiology are the
risk factors.* A striking feature of a risk factor
is that hardly anyone is concerned about its
proper definition.

Meijler notes that a report on the rationale of
the diet-heart statement by an AHA committee,
by S. M. Grundy, D. Bilheimer, and H. Blackburn,
et al, which appeared in *Circulation* in 1982, "fails
to define a risk factor though the term is used in
the text many times....*When a definition of risk
factor is given in a paper or a report, it often differs from the definition in another paper.*"

The Dutch cardiologist introduces a dash of
wry humor and reasons that, "When one takes these
definitions literally, one will soon notice that the
most obscure variables, such as the sale of nylon
stockings or the number of television sets, become
risk factors, as already suggested by Yudkin in
1957. Ideally, a factor should be called a risk factor only if, on elimination of that factor, the incidence of coronary heart disease would decrease."

The entire article is a well-reasoned, clear
presentation of facts in contrast to much of the
material on the subject. Dr. Meijler succinctly concludes:

"Considering the major risk factors linked with
coronary heart disease and the contribution of
their identification and modification to the care of
patients with coronary heart disease, we can only
conclude that their impact has been trivial."

If all the research and results of research on
risk factors has done little to help patients with
coronary heart disease – and the many other manifestations of atherosclerosis – why is this type of
research continued?

The answer, quite simply, is politics. When the boss has been successfully marketing apple pie for many years, it is politically unwise for an employee to advise the boss he would be more successful if he started marketing apple strudel.

Dr. Meijler closes his comprehensive paper with an amusing thought. "On the basis of these consideration it must be concluded that the contribution of risk factors to the daily care of patients with coronary heart disease is like an elephant that has delivered a mouse."

When the millions upon millions spent on risk factor research and the millions upon millions of lives which have not been saved by this research are considered, the concerns raised by scientists such as Meijler and Oster cannot be taken lightly.

Medical research, whether into cancer or atherosclerosis, unfortunately is vulnerable to the pressure of politics. And the politics of atherosclerosis, in turn, is vulnerable to the power of the dairy lobby.

The Milky Way

The dairy industry in America is large. The dairy lobby is one of the most powerful forces in Washington.   As reporter-editor William Robbins wrote, "...not even the International Telephone and Telegraph Corporation...could compare with the pervasive influence of a dairy lobby that represents one of the broadest reaches of power in the food industry."

Robbins adds, "Its purchases of political decisions and influence have been documented through court cases as well as through exposures resulting from scandals of the 1972 Presidential campaign, that dirtiest of all episodes ever studied by the Fair Campaign Practices Committee."

How does the dairy lobby acquire its influence? Giant combines like Associated Milk Producers, Inc., Mid-America Dairymen, Inc., and Dairymen, Inc., control 75 percent of America's milk production. All of the big milk co-ops are joined under the umbrella of the National Milk Producers Federation.

The dairy lobby spent almost half a million dollars in support of the Nixon campaign.

Contributions to other politicians, for their efforts in behalf of the dairy lobby, are also extensively documented.

Perhaps it is more germane to consider the influence the dairy lobby has on the public as a result of its advertising efforts. Americans have long been told that "Milk's a Natural." Everyone has heard that "milk is good for you." How accurate is this?

Aside from the XO threat milk poses, milk is also responsible for food allergy in children. Also, most of the world's adult population is intolerant of the sugar in milk called lactose which causes many people to have difficulty digesting milk. An overwhelming percentage of blacks and orientals are completely intolerant of lactose.

Oster has had several skirmishes with the National Dairy Council. In 1976, when the *National Enquirer* carried an *unsolicited* article by a freelance journalist on Oster's work, the Dairy Council sent out pamphlets to radio stations calling Oster a "publicity hound."

In actual fact, he had been approached by the writer who asked for an interview, saying that he hoped to sell the material to *Reader's Digest*. Much to Oster's surprise, the article came out in the *National Enquirer*, not the place Oster would ever have had considered suitable for his work. Later, when Oster was told that the Dairy Council had described him as a "publicity hound," he shrugged the matter off, knowing it was of little importance. However, the reaction of the Council was interesting. Oster explains,

"Early in 1983, I sent the National Dairy Council of America a copy of the research paper by Ross, Sharnick, and myself, 'Liposomes as a Proposed Vehicle for the Persorption of Bovine Xanthine Oxidase,' a rather technical article. As an example of the failure of the National Dairy Council to deal with the matter, Oster explains that, "the reply from the council stated that they would appreciate receiving 'research data, rather than opinion, in support of the hypothesis....' In this letter it also stated that we hadn't provided *any* evidence for our work.

"As can be seen from my response, I point out that the information in our paper is not opinion but research data."

March 3, 1983

M. F. Brink, Ph.D., President
National Dairy Council
6300 North River Road
Rosemont, Illinois 60018

Dear Doctor Brink:

I am in receipt of you letter of February 23....
First, the "Milk Fat Globules" report you sent
to me is old hat. It was described by S. Patton
and also is contained in Fundamentals of Dairy
Chemistry. It is completely irrelevant to our research because the fat globules described therein
come from raw milk, whereas our research deals
with liposomes created by the homogenization
process. These liposomes were manufactured
by the dairies and not by Ross et al, contrary to
your statement.

I quote as follows from our publication: Ross et
al, "Liposomes as a Proposed Vehicle for the Persorp-

tion of Bovine Xanthine Oxidase," Proc. Soc. Exp. Biol. & Med., Vol. 163, No. 1, January 1980:

> "In contrast to homogenized, pasteurized milk, raw milk contained only minute amounts of liposomes as demonstrated by measurement of enzyme activity and electron micrographic visualization." (Page 144)

I cannot understand how anyone can misunderstand this particular fundamental difference.

I also question your statement that stomach conditions with food should have a pH below 3.5. As stated in my publication in the Journal of the International Academy of Preventive Medicine, pages 43-46 (photocopy enclosed), your objection is dealt with by showing that the ingested milk buffers the gastric acidity. Even the research sponsored by you (Ho et al) admitted that. Our experimental conditions fully simulate natural processes found in human nutrition in contrast to the denatured product offered to the American youth.

Our research has been fully substantiated in a chapter of a forthcoming book published by Academic Press, New York, which will appear in June (of which I have a pre-publication copy). It confirms that liposomes in which xanthine oxidase is entrapped act as carriers of the enzyme through the body. Also, we did provide reference to the absorption of proteins through liposomes, which apparently is unknown to you, by quoting Dapergolas, F. et at, No. 17 reference in our publication, which should be readily available to you. I recommend you read this research to bring your knowledge up to date.

I am sorry that your connection with the National Dairy Council makes you stonewall actual data and refer to them as "opinions." The contrary research to our findings never has tried to duplicate our own experiments. I realize that the NDC supports Dr. J. Stamler's epidemiological research which, so far, has resulted in a fiasco as far as risk factor lowering is concerned; viz., the 115 million dollar debacle of MRFIT.

Sincerely yours,

Kurt A. Oster, M.D.

"What incentive does the National Dairy Council have to pay attention to our work?" asks Oster. Perhaps, it is the consumer who will call for change.

Experts Clash on Nutrition Policy

The medical community is all too uncomfortably aware of the differences in opinion when it comes to nutrition. Medical journals are a forum for the debate.

The *Journal of the AMA* published in 1979 an article headlined "Experts Clash On Nutrition Policy." In the opening lines, the statement that a "new national nutrition policy is struggling to be born" is amplified by the comment that "some would call the baby illegitimate."

The second paragraph of the article is equally pointed. "Researchers at the National Institutes of Health (NIH), where 11 separate institutes are now engaged in some form of nutrition research, are saying the nutrition debate is the most politicized issue ever to arise in the area of medical research."

Robert Edelman, M.D., of the National Institute of Allergy and Infectious Disease, is quoted in the *JAMA* article as saying that, "nutrition is the most politically charged area of science that I've ever seen."

The factions are very different and very opposed. In one camp there are individuals such as

Stanley Dudrick, M.D., chairman of the Department of Surgery at the University of Texas Medical School, Houston, stating that the lack of nutrition research is "one of the most shameful shortcomings of American medicine today."

In another camp there are groups such as the American Society for Clinical Nutrition (ASCN). Their task force published a comprehensive report that attempted to bring together for comparison and analysis the current scientific information on six dietary issues. This was done in an effort to help public officials establish a national nutrition policy for America. Incredibly enough, the report issued in May of 1979 by the ASCN was later "heartily disavowed by the same society."

Apparently, after the first precipitous groundswell of enthusiasm for a national nutrition policy, second thoughts surfaced.

Perhaps someone actually realized what an extraordinarily complex area nutrition is. Perhaps it was also realized that the political pressure was not going to help bring forth the best results. Certainly, the poor economic climate of the early 1980s worked against it. Funds were gradually reduced. Support was gradually withdrawn.

In June of 1981, the office of the Secretary of Agriculture announced that the Human Nutrition Center which produced the politically controversial "Dietary Guidelines for Americans" would be dismantled. Its divisions were to be redistributed to various agencies.

The dietary guidelines which had been issued in 1981 in collaboration with the Department of Health and Human Services had been heavily attacked by the meat and egg industries, and to a lesser extent by the dairy industry, for recommending that Americans avoid consuming "too much fat, saturated fat and cholesterol."

Yet misinformation on how eggs and other foods may increase serum cholesterol continues to be published, which means that studies in this area continue to be funded by the taxpayer.

Myth of the Healthy Savage

Enviably high on the *New York Times Book Review* nonfiction, best-seller list during the summer of 1981, and a strong seller for a long time after, was *The Pritikin Permanent Weight-Loss Manual*, described as a nutritionist's regimen for health and long life. It is a sequel to *The Pritikin Program for Diet & Exercise*, which sold over 400,000 in hardcover alone. Nathan Pritikin does well with the book extolling his diet. He also has several longevity centers.

The Pritikin diet has considerable appeal. The AMA Department of Foods and Nutrition commented in January 1980 that, "the Pritikin diet is promoted to the public as a regimen that can spare mankind much of the scourge of degenerative 'aging pathologies.' The diet is basically low in fats, (5% to 10% of total daily intake) and cholesterol (no more than 100 mg/day)...."

Because the general public in America has repeatedly been told that diets to lower fat and cholesterol intake are beneficial, the climate was favorable for acceptance by the general public.

How did Pritikin come up with his diet? Was it the product of many years of clinical testing? Close scrutiny reveals it is based on the diet of the Tarahumara (Flying Feet) Indians of north Mexico.

Pritikin does not have a medical background. But there are those in the American medical community who have studied the diet and lifestyle of these Indians and have been favorably impressed. Pritikin based the information in his books on the results of a nutritional survey of 372 Tarahumara in 1973 and 1974, published in the *American Journal of Clinical Nutrition* in April 1979. The conclusions of those conducting the survey was that the diet of the Tarahumara was "of generally high nutritional quality and would, by all criteria, be considered antiatherogenic." That is, the diet would not promote atherosclerosis.

Such a statement seems incentive enough to consider copying the diet of the Tarahumara as Pritikin has done. But there is more to the diet and lifestyle of these Indians than is revealed by those who extoll this tribe as a paradigm of good health because of sound nutrition.

Intrigued by all of the claims about the antiatherogenic diet of the Tarahumara, Oster decided to investigate further. What he uncovered was disappointing to say the least. A library search revealed a story by W.E. Garrett which was published in *National Geographic* in August 1968. As Oster flipped through the pages of this volume, the first photograph that caught his eye was of a spindly 14 pound two-year-old. The caption read: "Eighty percent of the Tarahumaras die before five of malnutrition or disease." Garrett reports in the article,

> ...the Tarahumaras live in the shadow of famine, despite efforts by Mexico's National Institute of Indian Affairs to improve their lot. They can coax only meager crops from the rocky soil. Though they herd cattle, sheep, and goats, and use the manure as fertilizer, they never milk the cows, and usually kill animals only for religious feasts.
>
> The Tarahumara live for the most part in the barren wilderness of the Sierra Madre Occidental. Their food comes from hunting and rudimentary agriculture.

Obtaining more information about this tribe Oster was amazed to discover that while the infant and child mortality rate for the average Indian tribe around the world is 50 percent, for the Tarahumara it is 80 percent.

"The Tarahumara are among the highest users in the world of peyote and mescaline. Their beer consumption is also considerable. About a hundred days annually are spent at beer parties and this beer supplies the Tarahumara with some ten percent of their dietary calories. Without the beer, their diet of eighty percent carbohydrates would be lethal. 'Witness the eighty percent mortality in Tarahumara children who eat the same diet but without beer'."

The Glory of the Long-Distance Runner

Much is made of the lean Tarahumara Indians' marathon running. It is frequently glorified. However, here again, the facts tell a different story. The July 1981 issue of *The American Medical Joggers Association Newsletter* states, "...Indians over 40 rarely take part in races and never train."

Natural History of January 1972 commented that, "The runners, jogging through darkness or through the heat of high noon, often chew peyote as a stimulant. At the end of the race sometimes only one man is left, the others having fallen away in exhaustion."

In June 1981, Oster wrote a letter to the *American Journal of Clinical Nutrition* in which he explained that although the "low level of serum cholesterol of the Tarahumara Indians is used extensively in the [medical] literature as an example of excellent dietary accomplishment," in his [Oster's] opinion, conflicting facts such as mortality rates and reports from other sources had not been sufficiently considered. Oster writes:

>I believe that the editors of *The American Journal of Clinical Nutrition* should have been provided with this evidence and should have informed their readers that this tribe, which has been quoted as a paragon of nutrition, actually is at the brink of famine and pays a frightful price to keep its plasma cholesterol low. I fear the so-called correlation of its plasma cholesterol value with its dietary cholesterol intake is an expression of the absolute minimum plasma cholesterol which may be reached before lack of resistance to disease and pathology develop. The low plasma cholesterol values of the Tarahamara should be considered an aberration of an insufficient diet and not as a norm to be emulated by followers of an unproved hypothesis. The oft reiterated statement that diets which result in a low plasma serum cholesterol will not cause any health damage, is again found wanting in one of nature's own experiments.

Oster's letter in the journal evoked a reply. One of the authors of a medical report on the Tarahumara of which Oster had been critical, sent an answering letter, explaining that "at no time have we ever suggested that Americans should adopt" the diet of the Tarahumara. But Pritikin did and continues to do so.

Among other details, the letter defended the medical report concerning the survey of the Tarahumara, noting that all of its "studies were centered around the village of Sisigouchi which is located in a very fertile valley. Corn and beans grow very nicely there and the soil is quite productive. The Tarahumara whom we studied were healthy individuals and were not starving. Our conclusion was that the Tarahumara diet was quite adequate nutritionally and, as used by the Tarahumaras, provided good nutrition which sustained their practice of long-distance running...."

The report on which Pritikin based his diet is

quite different from that of W.E. Garrett, who
called the Sierra Madre Occidental a land of "bar-
ren wilderness" which sustained only "meager
crops" because the medical survey was conducted
in only one village which was atypical of the whole
tribe. How representative would it be to prepare a
report about the state of health and nutrition in
the United States based on a survey of the healthy
residents of only one area. Perhaps Brooklyn, or
Harlem, or Scarsdale or Greenwich?

If the Tarahumara are truly outstanding in
their long-distance running ability, why haven't
they exhibited their prowess at the Olympics? Entry records reveal that although they have indeed
performed in some past Olympics, they don't seem
to be able to run so well away from home.

Various arguments have been offered to rationalize the poor performances of the Indians in
competition against runners from other countries,
ranging from the Tarahumara's lack of familiarity
with a runner's track and running shoes, and with
the high-protein diet fed them abroad.

The truth of the matter is that the Tarahumara's rocky, hilly terrain at home and their san-
dals, which consist of tire treads lashed to bare
feet with thongs, and their peyote and mescaline
habits would provide no edge over runners such as
Britan's Sebastian Coe and America's Steve Scott,
nor for that matter, over an average American col-
legiate runner. It is only because Olympic rules allow any nation to enter two competitors in an
event no matter what their qualifications that the
Tarahumara have appeared in the Olympics.

Can an average long-distance runner or a jogger benefit from adopting the Pritikin diet and perhaps improve performance time?

Apparently not. Contrary evidence is filtering
in that suggests the diet, which is imposed on the

Tarahumara by nature, may be outright dangerous for distance runners.

The July 1981 issue of *The American Medical Joggers Association Newsletter* contains a revealing editorial:

> When you hear about one of your friends being taken out of road racing because of a serious musculoskeletal injury CHECK HIS DI-ET! I've seen marathoners experiment with a low-fat or a vegetarian diet and then they vanish from the racing scene: groin pulls, torn Achilles' tendon, retinal detachment, fractures, back "injuries", etc. The first thing I [the author of the editorial] ask is about their intake of whole eggs, vitamin C and beer. MAGIC: If you find a runner who trains on a restricted diet and does not get injured, ask why. Often he has a supplement which makes the diet safe: wheat germ oil, yeast, nuts and seeds, etc. This isn't "magic" it is simple chemistry. EAT WHAT YOU CRAVE!
>
> For marathoners, the Pritikin diet or the "idealized Tarahumara diet" is dangerous because there isn't enough linoleic acid to protect cardiac function. Marathoners burn about 50 kcals of linoleic acid for each *mile* beyond the 20 km mark. Any diet with only 10% fat will have only 5% of the calories as linoleic acid... and remember that 5% of 2,000 kcals is only 100 kcals/day. If you burn fat and don't eat fat, you lose weight and your HDL goes down. But your HDL and your body fat can't go down forever; at some point you die a rhythm death — usually with a total cholesterol under 200 mg%.

The following extracts taken from the same newsletter should make distance runners, and indeed everybody, think twice about low-fat, low-cholesterol diets.

Dangerous Diet

> ...Tommy learned the idealized Tarahuma-
> ra diet from Pritikin; Dwyer learned it from
> Irwin Baker, who follows Pritikin, and the re-
> gression case actually used a "Tarahumara di-
> et" outlined by a nutritionist who has since
> moved away. (His cholesterol = 151 mg% at
> death!)
>
> All three avoided beer, megavitamin C,
> caffeine, animal fat, dairy products and eggs.
> All three used decaffeinated tea for fluid re-
> placement – avoiding beer. One added wheat
> bran to his food. CRAVINGS IGNORED: Beer
> is a great "thirst quencher" but "total absti-
> nence keeps my lipoprotein within control."

Diet Causes Runners to Die

The author of the Newsletter's editorial is a
qualified specialist whose unusual background results in his material offering a very unique viewpoint which is backed by hard facts. In the next
three cases he brings out facts which are rarely
identified by the average physician or a coroner
signing a death certificate.

> I predicted (*Atherosclerosis* 25:141, 1976)
> that 10,000 miles would improve angiograms.
> When the first cardiac patient showed this, I
> reported the improved angiograms (*Circulation*
> 61:666, 1980). However, 9 days before his
> death during sleep, he sat down and wrote me
> about this "great diet" he was on – his physi-
> cian did *not* know about the diet! I took the
> letter to the "death conference" and warned
> all the cardiac joggers to avoid the low-fat
> diet as soon as they reached the 10 k distance
> in rehab training. (Pritikin has also limited his
> in-house patients to 5 miles because of several
> episodes of arrhythmia when he combined 10 k
> distances with his low-fat diet).
>
> A cardiac marathoner [in San Diego] de-
> veloped osteoporosis of unknown cause. Multi-

ple fractures disabled him, but two long hospitalizations failed to uncover a cause. He died in his sleep. Ten years before he died he had recovered from a MI and began his rehab training. He finished 22 marathons and broke 3 hrs. The autopsy was normal except for an old healed MI and osteoporosis. I *predicted* that we would learn that he was on a low-fat diet; but it took us a while to check with his family. ANS: No supplemental vitamin C, no eggs, no whole milk, no red meat, no beer! In my view, the diet caused both the osteoporosis and the rhythm death. Bones require adequate protein, calcium and vitamin C. The heart requires adequate potassium, magnesium and EFA. Running increases your needs!

When I first saw the death certificate of Arne Richards, [of Kansas] I knew that it was wrong. It stated that he had died of acute myocardial infarction due to arteriosclerosis; but he was a lean marathoner who ran a good 50 kilometer race a week before he died. He never smoked. When I found his training partners they confirmed that he was "sort of a vegetarian... the *thinnest* marathoner in the area" and "drank a lot of tea." I *knew* this was another nutritional arrythmia. It took 18 months and I had to go to the Governor of the state to get an autopsy...and everything was normal. No disease! Nothing! Just a "rhythm death in a jogger." Tea has lots of phytates – blocks absorption of metals. Arne just did not have the nutrients he needed to train in the hot Kansas climate. He was 3 months away from his last sub-3-hour marathon – a former Editor of Runner's World – and a Professor of Library Science at the University of Kansas. Age 46.

This type of material takes us out of the realm of studying the *lifestyle* of individuals. The editor of the Newsletter explains that he works backwards from an autopsy, trying to find out what killed the runner. He warns: "If your serum cholesterol is less than 200 mg% you probably should not run marathons...see the six runners with low-cholesterol rhythm trouble in Cantwell's article in *Physician & Sportsmedicine* 9:69-82, 1981, March."

Oster once wrote to the editor of the *American Journal of Clinical Nutrition* that, "Generally speaking, defective scientific information may lead to false conclusions and costly and predictably unsuccessful experimentation, and contribute to the lack of credibility and disrepute of nutritional research." With regards to runners on the Pritikin-type, low-fat diet, "costly" translates into a very high price.

More Myths: The Masai of East Africa

One of Oster's recurring complaints about the hyperlipidemia theory is how much of it depends on epidemiology.

"There are liars, there are damn liars, and there are statisticians," he has been known to say. "But, don't get me wrong," as he roars with laughter. "My wife is an epidemiologist. One of the best, and epidemiology has its place in research."

"Study of related statistics have been invaluable to me on forging the connection between diet and atherosclerosis.

"Let me give you a practical example. When I first went looking for a possible dietary cause of atherosclerosis, I gathered statistics from around the world. I noted the consumption of milk, butter, and cheese in countries where such data was kept.

"Then I compared each population's death rate from atherosclerosis and degenerative heart disease with the consumption of dairy products.

"Homogenized milk consumption correlates to the incidence of atherosclerosis in every country.

"The pattern fit perfectly until I received information about the Masai of East Africa.

"These people didn't for some reason seem to fit the pattern. The Masai drink large quantities of milk, and the young warriors drink as much as seven liters per day which represents 60 percent of their calories as saturated fat. In spite of this, atherosclerosis is so rare among the Masai as to be almost nonexistent. You can be sure that I checked and rechecked the figures and the information carefully. But, there was apparently no mistake. Finally, because I had to have an answer, I personally went to East Africia in 1975.

"It took some time and it certainly didn't qualify as a sightseeing vacation, but I eventually uncovered a fascinating piece of information which had not previously appeared in any epidemiological data. Medical books which I had scanned also lacked this information.

"It became clear that the body of medical knowledge about the Masai was somewhat lopsided. It wasn't quite accurate.

"In scientific research a 'little bit wrong' is wrong!"

"The Masai do consume huge quantities of milk all right. *Curdled milk*, a type of yogurt...

"The difference between regular fluid milk and curdled milk has tremendous biological significance.

"Now we're talking about something quite different in their diet. Liquid milk is not the same type of food as the more solid, curdled milk. The former is rich in xanthine oxidase while the latter, as we and other researchers have shown, is practically devoid of biologically available XO. After I made this observation, the reason for the low rate of atherosclerosis among the Masai became obvious.

"If I had not been persistent enough (some say "stubborn") to travel to East Africa, this clarifcation of the facts might never have been made, and the bare statistics of epidemiology would have continued obscuring an important truth."

Fudging the Data

The following, from the film "Casablanca," usually brings a wry chuckle.

Rick (Bogart) "How can you close me up? On what grounds?"

Capt. Renault (Rains) "I'm shocked! Shocked to find that gambling is going on here."

Croupier, handing money to Renault "Your winnings, sir."

Renault, briskly "Oh, thank you very much."

Is it really funny to know that *authority* knows laws are flouted? Rather than weeping for lost innocence, one usually chooses to laugh at the cynicism of political expediency.

Are the politics of medicine so very different from the politics of any other group? Around the world, the medical community is charged with the ethical practice of medicine. Inevitably, political considerations must affect that charge.

Most people forget that no physician, whether general practitioner or specialist, could have treated human ills if medical research had not offered some solutions.

Without the legions of researchers and their fine work, physicians today might still have been helpless in the face of malaria, smallpox, syphilis, tuberculosis, cholera, scarlet fever; the list could run for pages.

Medical research has made bold and significant advances since the days when Servetus was burned to death for daring to cut up and examine the body of a dead man to further his knowledge of anatomy.

Whether the researchers have been loners like Semmelweiss or leaders like Pasteur, they did not work for prizes or for acclaim. Robert Koch, the physician-turned-bacteriologist, and Marie Sklodowska Curie, the chemist and physicist whose work twice merited the Nobel Prize, the first person to have achieved this honor, worked because they saw a need, they also believed they could help mankind.

Today, that same altruistic spirit is still a part of investigative medicine. Scientists still embark on voyages of discovery because, just possibility, their work might benefit humanity. Oster and Ross and others, such as Zikakis, have remained true to this tradition.

However, as unfortunate as it might be, the fine medical tradition has become tainted by those who view medicine as a vehicle for profit.

Early Warning Signals

Fudging the data is not the prerogative of individual researchers. Occasionally, the institution or the commercial enterprise for which the researcher works, manipulates research findings to suit its needs.

On April 17, 1983, the CBS-TV show, "Sixty Minutes," carried a story about Oraflex, a drug produced by Eli Lilly for arthritis relief.

In May of 1982, according to the "Sixty Minutes" report, Lilly sent 6,000 kits to television and radio news stations to promote the drug. Yet, for a least a year prior to this, Lilly researchers had apparantly known of Oroflex's serious side effects, which included death.

The drug was banned in September 1982 in the United Kingdom. A United States ban followed soon thereafter.

Michael Hensly, M.D., formerly an investigator for the Food and Drug Administration, spoke on the television show about the drug company's incomplete reporting of information to the FDA. He recommended "criminal prosecution of some Lilly employees for choosing not to submit research data."

Another disturbing case that blemished the medical profession concerned the heart stimulant drug, epinephrine. Its purpose is to revive patients' hearts after cardiac arrest, the drug is injected directly into the heart. Abbott Laboratories is one of the firms which commercially manufactures epinephrine.

Early in 1983, a paper in the *American Journal of Medicine* (*AJM*) offered a critical analysis of the Abbott drug's results. It suggested that the Abbott epinephrine, rather than being life-saving, may have actually been lethal. The co-authors of the article have a reputable collective background. Joseph Feldschuh, a physician for 21 years, is a cardiologist at both the New York Medical College and the New York Hospital Cornell Medical Center. Raymond Gambino, a Professor of Pathology at Columbia University is also president of Met Path Laboratories of Teterboro, New Jersey.

Shortly after the *AJM* report was published, Dan Dorfman's column in the New York *Daily News* covered the whole subject at some length. According to Dorfman the authors of the report in the *AJM* agreed to the Abbott officials' request that they omit certain information from their paper when the officials promised changes in the preparation of the drug. The information Feldschuh and Gambino had agreed to withhold was the 852 reported fatalities in 852 cases in which the drug had been administered!

In their report Feldschuh and Gambino suggest that among the million or so people who received Abbott's epinephrine injections, over a period of nine years, the survival rate was extremely poor.

What in Abbott's preparation caused their epinephrine to become lethal?

The Dorfman column explains that the Feldschuh-Gambino article in the *AJM* led to a warning about the drug's use from the Food and Drug Administration. And, in turn, Abbott, after a meeting with FDA officials, agreed to withdraw certain lots of the drug that were manufactured prior to July 1982.

> The article itself focused on just two deaths. But the background research (which Abbott was alerted to in June 1982) included reports of the 852 fatalities.
>
> In brief 38 physicians who had been surveyed on the use of the Abbott heart drug. In toto, 852 cases were cited where the patients had been treated with the Abbott epinephrine; and in every case the patient died.
>
> The Feldschuh-Gambino study, which was initiated by Feldschuh, arose after the heart specialist found an unusually high amount of acid in a patient who died in late '79. After discovering that the patient had been given Abbott's epinephrine, Feldschuh, later joined by Gambino, conducted in ('79 and '80) over, 1,000 biochemical tests of the product and two competing products (manufactured by Parke Davis and Bristol laboratories).

The findings: Abbott's drug contained 8.2 times the acidity of the Bristol product and 1,850 times the acidity of the Parke Davis heart drug. Epinephrine by itself is not acidic, but the solution, the vehicle in which it is contained, must be slightly acidic to preserve it.

The degree of acidity is measured by what's known as a pH valuation. The lower the pH reading, the higher the acidity. Human tissues have a relatively neutral pH value ranging between 7.38 and 7.42.

A person with a reading of pH 7 or less is considered to be in an extremely critical condition, since the acidity interferes with normal enzyme activity which brings life functions to a stop. The ultimate limit of survival is considered to be a pH of 6.85.

> The Feldschuh-Gambino study concluded overwhelmingly...that the Abbott epinephrine was lethal; that, once injected into a patient, it could lower the pH reading to as low as pH 6.
>
> Since Abbott has marketed millions of units of this drug (contained in syringes with accompanying needles) over the past nine years, Feldschuh contends, "Untold thousands may have died because this lethal drug gave the patients virtually no chance of resuscitation."
>
> In fact, in a letter he sent Feb. 1 to FDA Commissioner Arthur Hayes, sparked by his unhappiness over the FDA's "soft-pedaling" of a matter, Feldschuh's wrote, "A very real possibility exists that among the possible 1 million people; who may have received this injection over a nine-year period, that there may have been few, if any, survivors.
>
> ...the old Abbott epinephrine injected directly into the circulation as is usually the case, may be potentially lethal even to a healthy person.
>
> ...in his letter to the FDA, Feldschuh called on the agency to recall the current Abbott and Bristol preparations of epinephrine, as well as to set standards for all drugs.

If this medical reporting is accurate, the situation takes on the aspect of a holocaust. The saddening aspect of all this is what Feldschuh terms the FDA's "poor job" in response to the findings and their "failure to order a properly publicized recall of the drug" is inexcusable according to Feldschuh and Gambino.

One is puzzled how the FDA could have been so "soft," according to Feldschuh, in this matter; the same agency that continues to impose such tight restrictions on over-the-counter sales of folic acid, a non-toxic vitamin.

FDA Commissioner
Uneasy About Business Integrity

When the FDA is given information that is inadequate or incomplete, situations like those involving Oraflex or epinephrine result. This is not unique to the 1980s.

Dr. James L. Goddard, Commissioner of Food and Drugs some years ago, addressed the annual meeting of the Pharmaceutical Manufacturers Association in Florida in the spring of 1966. He told them he was "very uneasy about the way events are catching up with them."

> I will be quite candid with you: There is a real danger that the pharmaceutical industry as you and I know it today may be altered significantly, altered beyond your present fears, and altered beyond recall.
>
> If this sounds alarming, it is because − frankly − I am alarmed. Let me give you the basis for my feeling of alarm, after only 10 weeks in the Food and Drug Administration. During this brief but busy period I have seen evidence that too many drug manufacturers may well have obscured the prime mission of their industry: To help people get well.
>
> Let us agree that every industry has to make a profit for its stockholders. I am not against profit in the drug or any other indus-

try. The profit motive – as the Russians are finally discovering – stimulates beneficial activity: Competitive research and marketing, mass education, and the rise of the federal standard of living.

Gentlemen, we must keep our eyes on the patient. For – once you get through the medical reports and the counselors' opinions, the advertising and the marketing data, the licensing opinion, the advertising and the marketing data, the licensing and distribution agreements, the protocols and letter of credit, the labeling and packaging, and the report by the company treasurer   once you get through all that, you reach the physician who will administer your product to a human being.

At the end of the long line is a human life. Some of you seem to have forgotten this basic fact.

I cannot let you forget, as you cannot let me forget either. That is why I am genuinely concerned. Since becoming commissioner, I have come upon situations that I did not expect. I know that many of you, were you to sit in my chair for a week, would be as troubled as I. Therefore, I am bringing to your attention some things that you must be aware of, for only you know how to correct them.

Problem of Dishonesty

In addition to the problem of quality, there is the problem of dishonesty in the investigational drug stage.

...Now, I will admit that Government employes do not have a corner on all wisdom. And I will admit that there are gray areas in the I.N.D. [Investigator's New Drug] situation.

But the conscious withholding of unfavorable animal or clinical data is not a gray-area matter.

...The planting in journals of articles that begin to commercialize what is still an investigational new drug is not a gray-area matter.

These actions run counter to the law and the ethics governing the drug industry.

Let us move on to new drug applications. This is the take-off stage, as you know, for a new product of this industry. Now we must review the clinical evidence, the labeling and advertising, the promotional materials, package inserts – you are as familiar with the process as I.

...I have been shocked at the materials that come in to us. I have been shocked at the clear attempts to slip something by us. I am deeply disturbed at the constant, direct, personal pressure some industry representatives have placed upon our people. Gentlemen, the N.D.A. situation needs your attention – and now.

...Government alone cannot serve all the health needs of the American people. This is a responsibility we gladly share with private industry.

But you cannot accept the partnership lightly.

The FDA and their work with drug manufacturers is only one part of the picture.

Venture into the arena of medical research and you have entered a complex place. It is a labyrinth difficult to follow even for those of its members who are knowledgeable in its ways.

The High and Mighty Tainted

The disquieting news of scientists faking research data and results made headlines with alarming frequency in the 1980s.

"U.S. to Penalize Heart Researcher on Fraudulent project at Harvard," headlined the *New York Times*, February 16, 1983.

Yale, Cornell, Harvard, Boston University, Sloan-Kettering, Mount Sinai, these and other distinguished medical institutions have all uncovered bizarre episodes of scientific misconduct, or "drylabbing it," as scientists term the work of colleagues whose facts come from their imaginations and not from their laboratories.

A year-long investigation by the National Institutes of Health centered on the falsification of papers published by a Harvard Medical School scientist. The "scientific audit...shook the research community, overturned promising careers and started an agonizing re-evaluation of the scientific method."

The NIH censured the school's laboratory procedures and supervision and asked for repayment to the U.S. Government for one project on which data was falsified.

The scientist was barred from receiving Federal funds for a decade. If this seems a mild penalty, consider that in the past, researchers who had *admitted* to fraud could *continue* to receive Federal funds.

The *New York Times* explained in a March 1983 article, "for the first time in the annals of scientific crime, the Federal Government recently blamed a case of fraud not only on the perpetrator but on the society in which he worked...."

Ultimately, large amounts of material in at least five Harvard research projects, all animal studies, were found to have been falsified by the accused scientist, an apparently promising 31-year-old cardiologist. The bogus information found its way into nine co-authored published papers and numerous extracts. Even previous work by the cheating scientist came under scrutiny and was found wanting.

At Harvard, it was cardiac work with dogs that eventually aroused suspicion. A researcher noticed that a chart purported to show facts and figures of work on a single animal, without interruption, over 24 hours, 48 hours, 72 hours, and seven days. He concluded that it was "highly unlikely" that the recording apparatus had not been used for any other studies during that entire week.

When the cardiologist claimed to have done autopsy work on the dog's heart, the body, with heart intact, was produced. Suspicious co-workers had recovered the body of the dog and had saved it for evidence.

When accusations were leveled at the scientist, one more transgression came to the surface. The man had unaccountably thrown away notebooks and information on much of the work under question. Clearly, he'd broken a major rule of research, that all documentation is scrupulously preserved. Eventually, the accusations of forgery and cheating were proved.

The Harvard situation, more than most other cases of research fraud, raises the issue of "whether something in the highly competitive research enterprise, some flaw in the system, pushes talented scientists to cheat, gives them too much opportunity to do so, and makes it fiendishly difficult to uncover the extent of it when it occurs," said Dr. Howard E. Morgan, chairman of the Federal panel that investigated Harvard. The chairman added, "...there is intense pressure to publish. The system of science today demands visible evidence of success. In its absence, universities will deny a scientist tenure and the Government will cut off grants and contracts.

"Sometimes the pressure put on the major figures of medical research are enormous."

Are these mounting pressures fueled by the infighting for Federal funds? Perhaps researchers stand a better chance for recognition when they know their projects fall comfortably within established guidelines.

Perhaps this is why few have dared to support Oster and Ross openly. Interestingly, in private, communications researchers from reputable universities have expressed to Oster their support of his ideas. Publicly, these voices remain muted because of politics.

Riddled With Doubt

The serious question of how much data is bogus is overshadowed by the ultimate query: Why?

"Where does the problem lie?" questioned an article in the *Journal of the American Medical Association* in its April 8, 1983 issue.

Is "something inherently wrong in the system, the person, or both, that allows such behavior to emerge," mused Eugene Braunwald, M.D., one of America's top cardiologists and a member of the National Academy of Sciences. Dr. Braunwald was the senior scientist in the Harvard situation, which drew particular attention to the relationship between senior and junior scientists, the "master-apprentice bond pivotal to scientific progress since the days of Plato and Pythagoras."

Strain in the balance between senior and junior scientist, teacher and student, is serious. In the past few decades, "the balance has sometimes been thrown out of whack, in part because the scientific enterprise in post-war America has grown large and affluent. Its hallmark has become the laboratory chief who builds an empire and rules from afar."

According to the *New York Times* article, "while his protégé forged data, Dr. Braunwald was busy as physician-in-chief to Brigham and Women's Hospital and Beth Israel Hospital, both Harvard affiliates in Boston; head of two laboratories; director of nearly a score of scientists, and fiscal overlord of at least 3.3 million in Federal research funds."

The budgets for research projects are large,

and growing. So are the pressures. The resulting problems of fraud have surfaced in all the fields of medical research.

The Patchwork Mouse, by Joseph Hixon, was published in 1976. It is about "politics and intrigue in the campaign to conquer cancer," the $1.7 billion campaign that President Richard Nixon and the Congress of the United States began in 1970.

Joseph Hixon, a veteran medical science reporter, examined the ambitions of research scientists – and the scandal of investigators who operate "in a climate of high rewards and strong temptations."

The Sloan-Kettering Institute for Cancer Research in New York City was embroiled in charges that its director Robert Good had turned one of his many young protégés loose and "told anyone who would listen that the young researcher seemed to have made an important breakthrough."

A breakthrough was deliberately faked, one that was supposedly able to prevent the rejection of organ transplants in mice. A young researcher had painted the fur of experimental mice with a marking pen to make it appear that the organ transplants had been successful.

It was said about Good's protégé that "it was the pressure to produce results... that drove him to commit the unpardonable sin of science, faking test results."

"I don't go along with the idea that if you're under pressure, it's an excuse for cheating," Thomas C. Chalmers, M.D., Dean of Mount Sinai School of Medicine in New York, reported in JAMA "Cheating is not just an abrupt and isolated phenomenon in research, it's on the end of a slope.... We have created a milieu in which absolute honesty is not the be-all and end-all."

Which Institution Has Status?

Who makes the decisions about which researchers receive grants? For the most part, this is
entrusted to committees of scientific experts, the
peer-review system. Almost invariably, committee
members come from the same elite institutions
that win most grants.

Oster's collaborator, Dr. Ross, points out that
in America status wins points. The elitist attitude
breeds a prejudice against relatively unknown individuals such as Oster and Ross, whose tie to the
academic world is Fairfield University. Fairfield,
founded in 1942 is relatively young and small. The
new priesthood of internationally recognized researchers from Harvard, or Yale, or MIT hardly expect anything good to come from Fairfield.

"Where's that? What could they think of that
we haven't?"

Also, the referee system is the precaution a-
gainst fraud. This means that almost all scientific
journals send out the manuscripts they receive for
publication to experts, whose task is to catch de-
fects in argument or in technique.   Unfortunately,
analysis shows that "refereeing is more susceptible
to bias than peer review." In one study, 10 high-
quality published articles were resubmitted to the
very same journals that had published them several years earlier.   The authors' real and sometimes
prestigious names and affiliations were replaced
with fictitious ones. The second time around only
four of 22 reviewers recommended publication.

The inbred quality of the system and its element of inherent bias can be tacitly ignored by the
scientific community because they know they have
an ultimate safeguard.   The final and formidable
defense against inaccurate or fraudulent scientific
work is repeatability.

Scientists are supposed to describe exactly how they did their experiments so that others can repeat the work and either confirm or refute results.

The truth is that scientists rarely bother to repeat one another's experiments because replication of others findings does not lead to recognition or to grant awards. Reports are often therefore accepted at face value. This, however, has not been the case with the work of Oster and Ross. The research involving XO has not been accepted at face value, although a handful of reputable scientists have looked at the work with genuine objectivity.

In December 1974, the Food and Drug Administration asked the Life Sciences Research Office of the Federation of American Societies for Experimental Biology (FASEB) to prepare a review of Oster's work. Ross calls the 65-page document "fair."

"The FASEB review suggested a number of useful approaches to increasing out knowledge in this area," Ross acknowledges.

"In essence, the report says, 'Yes, we see what you've done. We'd like to see the results of other researchers in this field. The work does merit further investigation'."

Ross adds that, "Now, almost a decade later, Oster and I can point to the experimentation of other scientists whose research on XO corroborates ours.

"Repeatability lends respectability," Ross emphasizes. "When you publish your work, you hope to stimulate others to explore its boundaries, push them even further. This both confirms your work and helps expand knowledge in the field. But repeating experiments takes time and money. The rewards are few.

"Despite this, our work has succeeded in stirring the imaginations of a select few, independent scientists interested in our field. The first two papers Oster and I published stimulated Dr. Zikakis of the University of Delaware. A number of his experiments confirmed ours. For instance, he fed XO to experimental animals then measured antibodies to the XO in their bodies. He then extended that antibody study to large numbers of people.

"The work by Zikakis, in turn, drew a response from Dr. Helion Povoa of the University of Rio de Janeiro Medical School. He actually flew up to visit Oster. Povoa's work is mainly on plasmalogen. He found that injecting XO in experimental animals depleted plasmalogen in arterial tissue. He also found that folic acid may restore plasmalogen.

"The obvious conclusion is that folic acid does favor the synthesis of plasmalogen. Povoa could actually regulate the level of plasmalogen in artery walls by administering folic acid.

"Such results lend respectability to our work.

"An extensive body of scientific and medical literature supports the various aspects of our work. In 1925, O. M. Schloss made a comprehensive review of research dating back to 1844 which dealt with the absorption of whole undigested milk proteins. Dr. K. Isselbacher et al. have investigated the absorption of undigested macromolecules and have shown that large molecules can indeed cross the intestinal wall. J. R. Davies et al. of Wales have demonstrated the presence of antibodies to cow's milk proteins (not specifically to bovine xanthine oxidase as we have done) in coronary heart disease patients and found significantly higher antibody levels in those patients with coronary heart disease.

"G. R. Greenbank and M. Pallansch published in 1962 their observation that 'pasteurization of milk as it is done in the United States leaves approximately 42 percent of the xanthine oxidase intact and in its active state'.

"In 1953, the *Quarterly Review of Pediatrics* presented the paper from a Symposium on Homogenized Vitamin D Milk and Human Health. The article by F. J. Doan, Professor of Dairy Science, the Pennsylvania Agricultural Experiment Station, State College, Pennsylvania, explains that when milk is homogenized, the fat globules are reduced in size by at least 3.5 times their original dimension."

Ross adds that "as a result of this unnatural micronization, the number of fat globules is increased producing an expansion of the fat globule surface for the absorption of XO. As a result, the biological availability of XO is multiplied by at least a factor of 3.5. This increases XO's potential for absorption through the intestinal mucosa undigested; it eventually reaches the bloodstream via the lymph system and is deposited ectopically...in the heart muscle and the arterial wall."

The research Ross has been conducting with Oster has spanned over a decade. Thus, he is one of the world's leading authorities on the XO topic. He is articulate and quite adept at explaining the subject to the uninitiated. He is confident that, with time, new researchers will further substantiate and expand on what he and Oster have uncovered. Even so, Ross cannot help but feel frustrated.

"Virtually nothing is being done today about the menace of homogenized milk. The connection between XO and atherosclerosis is being ignored. That is very difficult to accept. I hope that public awareness of this will soon change."

Prevention of Atherosclerosis: Fact or Fiction

Oster, by virtue of his experience, analyzes

the issues that confront medical researchers with a keen eye. He has published and lectured extensively about the controversy that surrounds the possible causes of atherosclerosis. However, because such arguments are usually found only in scientific journals, most people are not aware of the heated debate waged in the medical arena.

As an outspoken critic of those who insist saturated fat and cholesterol are responsible for atherogenesis, one of the most significant papers Oster has published concerning the controversy is titled "Prevention of Atherosclerosis: Fact or Fiction? A Critique of the Report of the Inter-Society Commission for Heart Disease," which was published in the April 1972 issue of *Medical Counterpoint*.

The report that Oster reviews in his article is the "Primary Prevention of the Atherosclerotic Disease." It appeared in a 1970 issue of *Circulation*. At the start of Oster's ten-page critique, the editor of *Medical Counterpoint* states:

> EDITOR'S NOTE: Dr. Oster's paper takes issue with certain conclusions of the Inter-Society Commission Report that have been drawn from the Framingham Study concerning the risk of coronary heart disease. It particularly challenges the stated relative effect on risk of CHD at different levels of serum cholesterol. Some of the questioning is based on clinical experience confirmed by others (e.g., the unimportant effect on serum cholesterol levels of significant reduction in dietary cholesterol).
> In December 1970, The Inter-Society Commission for Heart Disease Resources, "comprised of outstanding leaders in the field of cardiovascular diseases and representatives of national professional organizations capable of making significant contribution," reported its suggestions for the prevention of atherosclero-

tic diseases.

In its introductory note to the reader, the Commission invites constructive criticism of the work of its study groups, particularly those who attempt to apply these guidelines. In the following paper such constructive criticism will be given and it will be shown that the Report of the Commission is prejudicial, based on dubious data and therefore probably deceptive. Furthermore, by thus wasting the taxpayers' money, the Report of the Commission, instead of advancing the cause of coronary heart disease prevention, channels the research funds overwhelmingly into narrow, preconceived, subjective, discredited areas of research. It thereby hinders, if it does not preclude, the development of other approaches which may provide more effective solutions of this problem, so vital to the health of the American people.

To the tune of scheduled press conferences and through recourse to the various media, the American people were advised to change their diets drastically and especially curtail the consumption of cholesterol to 300 mg daily from the usual 600 mg and to reduce the intake of saturated fats to 35% from 40%. Admittingly having no proof on which to base these revolutionary recommendations that would affect the life habits of the American people and alter the manufacturing of basic foods and the raising of livestock, the Commission presents some alleged facts, studies, and tables to support their unproven theories.

A questionable transformation takes place by semantic legerdemain on the part of the Commission. The risk of coronary heart disease in 92 persons out of a group of 1329 reported by Cornfield is equated by the Commission to the incidence of coronary heart disease in many millions of the U.S., if not the world's population − a subsitution which is unacceptable. Again, we doubt the accuracy of the data presented to the computer.

One of the most valuable jobs Oster performs for the general reader is to bring some perspective to the previous remarks and attitudes of those who produce official reports such as this. The fifth page of Oster's review carries the information that:

> Cornfield must have sensed these short-comings because in a later (1969) publication he stated, "We must admit at the outset that we have no secure basis for estimating the reduction in incidence of or mortality from coronary heart disease that could be achieved by application of current knowlege." He also states in the same article, "It seems clear that despite a very considerable scientific effort and some tantalizingly suggestive results, we have no clear-cut generally accepted answer to the question whether cholesterol lowering measures can affect coronary heart disease." We concur in Cornfield's doubts. We feel that his equation is not valid biologically and should not be used to substantiate the implied effect of proposed dietary changes suggested by the Commission.

What the report doesn't say is almost as important as what is does say. Oster expands upon this idea in his critique:

> Furthermore, the statement of Pearce and Dayton, [10] who warn that their findings are not to be construed as recommending a change in the American diet, are alarmingly absent in the Commission's Report. The fact that there is a potential danger from unsaturated fatty acids as carcinogenic agents is underplayed. The American people are led to believe that unsaturated fatty acids do not undergo chemical changes under heating and during cooking though such changes are a fact well known to every organic chemist but not mentioned in the Inter-Society Commission Report.
> If publications of the individual members

constituting the Commission are examined, one finds that in July, 1970 J. T. Doyle wrote in an editorial in the *Annals of Internal Medicine*, [11] about the prevention of coronary heart disease: "The conscientious physician must then be guided by his instincts, his common sense, and the fundamental principle that he should do no harm." In December of the same year, one finds him as a member of the Commission giving his consent to sweeping recommendations of dietary changes.

A more cautious view of such dietary change is reflected in the remarks of Dr. Donald S. Frederickson when discussing the Inter-Society Commission Report in his St. Cyres Lecture of the National Heart Hospital at the Royal College of Physicians of London, published in the British Medical Journal:[12]

"There are some things about the report to be pitied, however. In the light of what is actually known, the injuctions on consumption of cholesterol and fats seems too radical as they stand. What evidence do we have that an egg yolk a day spells jeopardy for all Americans?

"...One looks vainly in the Commission Report for something new and strong enough to change the present governmental non-position concerning dietary fat consumption..."

The Commission disregards the potential economic dislocations which would result from their recommendations, should they become reality. It also completely disregards the warnings and excellent deliberations in the Report of the Diet-Heart Review Panel of the National Heart Institute (dated June 1969 and published as American Heart Association Monograph No. 28, 1969, which antedates the Inter-Society Commission Report). The members of that panel have at least the same scientific standing and authority, but act more responsibly than the members of the Inter-Society Commission.

By critical analysis of the Report of the Inter-Society Commission for Heart Disease Resources concerning the prevention of ather-

osclerosis, one is led to endorse the opinions of
Ludwig and Collette: [13] "Errors of presentation include improper generalizations and the
incautious use of secondhand data." We feel
that the Commission presented its findings in
a misleading manner.

We quote again from Ludwig and Collette,
"More serious consequences follow when erroneous conclusions are drawn from invalid data or through faulty or incomplete analysis.
Health programs may be augmented or discontinued, health practices modified, and worth-
less solutions to health problems advanced, all
on the basis of misinformation."

Scientific Addition and Subtraction

One interesting aspect of the critique by Oster
is a review of *his* analysis of the Inter-Society
Commission Report by the counsulting mathematician Stephen A. Bauman. As an impartial third party, Bauman raises points that reinforce Oster's al-
legation that many of the conclusions drawn from
the MRFIT and Framingham studies are invalid.

The mathematician is careful to remain the
impartial observer, one who uses his technical
skills to expose flaws in reasoning and inaccuracies
in conclusions. As objective as the mathematician
is, he points out the difficulty, if not the impossi-
bility, of arriving at truly accurate information
with the methods used by the Inter-Society Commission.

As Oster point out, this is all the more reason
to refrain from making dietary recommendations
on the basis of the Inter-Society Commission Report.

In his critique, Bauman refers to the Commission's report with words which include, "guessed"
and "assumption."   He also states that certain
claims in the Commission's paper make "no valid

comparisons" and that "These ranges do not constitute discrete thresholds for risk."

The conclusion of the mathematician's review is telling: "One must be careful to differentiate between risks for different populations and cause/effect. Statistical studies of population samples, such as the Framingham Study, cannot show *how* a reduction in an individual's serum choleterol level would affect his risk of CHD. These studies are designed to suggest areas for further research. As a result of this initial study, additional parameters were examined at Framingham."

Did anyone remind the medical researchers to be careful to differentiate between risks for different populations and for cause/effect?

Room for Rebuttal

The credentials of both Oster Kurt A. Oster and his colleague Donald J. Ross are impeccable. Independent researchers around the world have corroborated much of the experimentation Ross has done at Fairfield University.

Nevertheless, Oster's work lacks official support. Indeed, he has gathered his fair share of criticism. He has been consistently denied a hearing at American Medical Association conferences despite the fact that his work has been published in reputable scientific journals.

In 1970 Oster started corresponding with Connecticut Senator Ribicoff who saw to it that Oster could have a hearing before the National Institutes of Health, in Bethesda, Maryland. Oster thus had an opportunity to present his research findings to Dr. Theodore Cooper, who at that time was the Director of the Heart and Lung Institute (later Dr. Cooper, as the Assistant Secretary of Health, personally injected President Ford with the notorious swine flu vaccine, an event receiving national press coverage).

Not until a few years after his trip to Bethesda did Oster fully comprehend why his two-hour presentation to the NIH group on XO had evoked only lackluster interest. The people at the Heart and Lung Institute had apparently already committed themselves to the MRFIT program. "What I had to say about XO fell on deaf ears." Oster and Ross have not lost faith over the years.

"My opponents describe me as friendly and sincere," Oster chuckles grimly as he repeats the words.

"I've been told I'm a warm, likable fellow with an honest manner. But I'm also persistent and if no one else will act on the results of my scientific work, I will not give up and be quiet. People die of atherosclerosis. We have a way to help. I want people to be aware of how they can be helped. That's one of the reasons I've taken the time and trouble to work on a book like this. It's very important for people to understand why much of the criticism of my work is inaccurate."

Detractors of Oster's work often seem guilty of faulty scientific and medical judgments. Occasionally, they even seem to be ignorant of the facts. Over the years, Oster and Ross have published numerous rebuttals of criticisms leveled against their work.

Early in 1982, Oster was asked by the editors of the *Swedish Journal of Biological Medicine* to write an article about his work. He was also asked to include his analysis of criticism by his opponents.

The article that Oster wrote for the Swedish journal is a fascinating account of his work and the scientific verification of his original concept. The labor of more than four decades is neatly presented in a careful, precise manner. "Reflections on a Dietary Cause of Atherosclerosis and on its Opponents," which was published in the September issue of the Swedish journal, is reprinted in the appendix. Highlights from the article are given below.

When an archaeologist attempts to restore structures of earlier times, his main concern is finding the cause of the destruction of the underlying formations and to rebuild those original forms. He is aided in this enterprise by the discovery of bits and pieces of the structures, shards, coins, and other artifacts. He is less interested in the origin or composition of the superficial layer of dust and debris which, over the centuries, have accumulated and have shielded the underlying relics from discovery.

An analogy can be made with the lesions of atherosclerosis. For the past thirty years, research has been concerned with the origin of the covering of the original injury to the arterial wall. Most researchers have an unhealthy preoccupation with the deposited layers of cholesterol, fibrin, and calcium. They postulate that by lowering serum cholesterol, one not only prevents further deposition of cholesterol but also removes that which is already present, and that by removing these manifestations of the natural healing process, one might then remedy the consequences of the original injury. This approach has not affected greater cardiovascular health, despite the expenditure of billions of scarce research dollars.

In order to understand the development of any pathological reaction, one should have a solid knowlege of the original basic structures. Without this information, scientific endeavor will degenerate to investigations of association, of circumstantial evidence leading to speculations and exercises in numerology which are given the impressive name of "risk factor".

In his article, Oster notes that some of the objections to his work are based on outdated information. More than one researcher has relied on discredited information.

A researcher at the National Institutes of Health, as well as researchers sponsored by the dairy industry, have stated that Oster's conviction that XO in cow's milk can be absorbed by the body is wrong. In a letter to Oster a NIH researcher made reference to an outdated textbook and stated that XO ingested in milk is destroyed by gastric acidity and intestinal enzymes and that, in addition, the large molecular size of XO precludes its passage through the intestinal barrier.

"Those who continue to perpetuate such assumptions expose an Achilles' heel," chuckles Oster.

"The basis on which this criticism is made cannot be any more wrong. These critics neglect to consider that much of the xanthine oxidase which is consumed in liquid milk is not destroyed because milk is a powerful buffer which can neutralize gastric acidity. Furthermore, the homogenization process creates the new physical entities known as 'liposomes' which sequester XO and enable most of it to be carried past gastic juices and pancreatic enzymes undigested."

The research of G. Gregoriadis has established that a similar "protective influence" by liposomes keeps insulin from being digested when it is ingested orally by diabetics. Thus insulin can be absorbed more effectively from the intestine. A number of pharmaceutical companies are now employing liposomes to facilitate passage of a digestible drug, or hormone, across the intestinal barrier.

In 1965 Al-Khalidi and his research team tested the serum of 40 human volunteers and found no XO. In 1976 McCarthy and Long found no XO activity in the serum of milk-fed pigs. Opponents of Oster utilize such findings to support their contention that XO cannot enter the circulation intact. On the surface this argument may seem valid. However, it is a premature conclusion which reflects pedestrian thinking. It overlooks the critical point that XO is hidden in liposomes. "Free-floating" XO is not present in blood serum, so attempts to find it in this form have been fruitless.

Oster explains that his work with Ross has shed light on the fate of XO after it traverses the intestinal barrier into the circulation:

> We could not demonstrate any xanthine oxidase activity in normal human serum either before or after milk consumption...subsequently, we discovered the enzyme sequestered in liposomal form following milk consumption.
>
> The simplistic idea...that ingestion of xanthine oxidase in homogenized milk should lead to its demonstrable presence in human serum and that its absence from serum is proof of its non-absorption is, biologically speaking, both naive and untenable. Any absorbed circulating xanthine oxidase would be destroyed by passage of the blood through the liver filter.
>
> These artificially created vesicles (liposomes) attach themselves to, or are ingested into white blood cells and can be chemically demonstrated there. This affinity for white blood cells is how liposomes avoid destruction by liver reticulocytes and how liposomal content, such as xanthine oxidase, may be carried to...arterial walls and heart muscle and deposited there. Once ensconced in a foreign or ectopic location, the enzyme exerts its action on the membranes of the cells surrounding it.

In Oster's opinion, work by Ho and Cifford of the University of California at Davis, which was sponsored by the National Dairy Council and which attempts to refute his findings, must be considered with great care. Oster agrees with the concerns expressed in an article in the *New York Times,* December 3, 1980, over the fact that research can be influenced by its financial underwriters. Oster and Ross don't understand how Ho and Clifford can, after conceding on the basis of their experimentation that small quantities of XO do enter the circulaton intact, conclude that the absorbed XO has no biological significance.

Writing in the *Swedish Journal of Biological Medicine*, 1982, Oster takes direct aim at those who attempt to discredit his work with sketchy evidence while ignoring the intricacies of the XO-plasmalogen disease mechanism.

> Xanthine oxidase will specifically destroy plasmalogen contained in the cell membrane, most probably by the creation of superoxides which are not vulnerable to the influence of serum superoxide dismutase. As a result, the cells so affected can react to this membrane damage by proliferation and eventual necrosis. Thus is created a primary injury which can be repaired according to local conditions. Repair of damage to arterial structures is mostly accomplished by introduction and deposition of cholesterol esters, fibrin, and disintegration material of thrombocytes; injury of the myocardium heals with connective scar tissue formation.
>
> These intricate biological findings have been ignored by the National Dairy Council sponsored work of Ho and Clifford in Davis, California.
>
> In contrast to Ghandi and Ahuja, Ho and Clifford were unable to determine intravenously administered xanthine oxidase in the myocardium of rabbits. They also claim that xanthine oxidase administration did not deplete the heart or aorta of plasmalogen, again contradicting the results of Ghandi and Ahuja. An examination of the reported results of Ho

> and Clifford leaves their methodology and conclusion open to serious doubts because of the small number of animals employed in each experimental category (average three or less) and the wide variations of the standard errors.
>
> Another inept attempt to criticize the BMXO concept was the inappropriate methodology by Volp and Lage to exclude persorption of a large protein molecule. Their method was never designed to attack this problem.

Referring to a comprehensive review of his work by H. C. Deeths, a research chemist for the Australian dairy industry, which was published in the *Journal of Dairy Science*, July 1983, Oster points out that his dairy sponsored opponents have changed their tune of late. No longer is the claim being made that all XO is digested and rendered inactive in the stomach. Quoting from Deeth's paper: *"Biologically available XO in consumed milk products may be absorbed in the small intestine and enter the bloodstream."* (emphasis added).

Somehow the conclusion is drawn by Deeths that "there appears to be no unequivocable evidence that the absorbed enzyme has any pathological effects that may contribute to the development of atherosclerotic heart disease."

Oster chuckles, "after billions of dollars on cholesterol research there is *no unequivocable* evidence that dietary cholesterol triggers atherosclerosis either."

One of the main objections to the BMXO work centers around the fact that the human liver and certain parts of the intestine contain xanthine oxidase. Critics of Oster's work state that XO found in arterial tissues might come from these sources.

Oster replies, "These objections defy simple logic and the rules of fundamental immunology."

He explains that, "specific antibodies are derived in man when xenobiological (foreign) proteins

are introduced to the immune system. The xanthine oxidase which triggers an antibody response
in the body must come from an outside source.

"Al-Khalidi found clinically significant human
xanthine oxidase in the bloodstream of patients
with liver disease. If the xanthine oxidase found in
human arterial wall lesions would be of human origin, we would have to conclude that atherosclerosis
is the result of liver disease. An unlikely assumption, at best."

Recently, Oster was encouraged when Bierman
and Shank of the Committee of Nutrition of the
American Heart Association alleged they would be
conducting research into his work. However, instead of the promised research, Bierman and Shank
merely wrote an editorial in which they raised theoretical objections to his work. Thus, once again,
Oster found himself having to enlighten the "high
and mighty." He took the opportunity to bring some
facts into focus in the Swedish journal.

> A JAMA editorial [24] written by the
> chairman of the American Heart Association
> Committee on Nutrition also mistakenly
> equates my biochemical concept of athero-
> sclerosis with causes of coronary heart disease.
> ...The authors do not seem to understand
> that coronary artery diesease is but one mani-
> festation of the complex of atherosclerotic
> diseases.
> I consider Bierman and Shank's statement
> that the hypothesis has been stated and re-
> stated by a single protagonist as an honorable
> position, not a detraction. Historic prece-
> dence has been set by other scientists who
> were found to be right after the establishment
> fought them and their positions. Furthermore,
> most of the objections raised by Bierman and
> Shank .have been overcome by further confirm-
> ing experimentation, [5,12,27] making the sin-

gle protagonist issue no longer tenable.

The xanthine oxidase concept approaches the cholesterol question from a biochemical angle, since it cannot be denied that high levels of serum cholesterol in man are associated with increased severity of atherosclerotic diseases.

Other biological sterols, as the male hormone anderosterol and vitamin D, are also promoters of the atherosclerotic process [32]. Many of these substances stimulate xanthine oxidase activity.

Soup Anyone?

Fortunately, Oster's sense of humor and his sense of the absurd rarely desert him. In the 1970s, he demonstrated an important point in support of his work in a somewhat wicked way at a meeting of the International Academy of Preventive Medicine.

When Oster and Ross initially set off on their journey into the unpredictable world of medical research, they took for granted many things that had been taught to them in textbooks. As they got deeper into their own trailblazing efforts, they found themselves producing results not found in textbooks. Ross, for instance, was highly skeptical when Oster suggested he might find a milk enzyme in an arterial wall. Ross had been taught what all physicians had been taught — that the human body digests all proteins to amino acids, so that no complex protein is absorbed into the body.

Then, to his surprise, when Ross reviewed the literature, he found that as far back as 1911 Schloss had reviewed a body of work showing many instances in which undigested proteins may pass through the intestinal wall. Somehow, these citations had never made it into medical textbooks.

It is not surprising that when Oster and Ross announced that they were finding XO antibodies in the bloodstream, their fellow scientists resisted the idea.

Yet, it is undeniable that occasionally harmful protein molecules do get into the body.

For instance, there is botulism.

When food is tainted with Botulinus toxin, which happens to be a larger protein than XO, and a person ingests the toxin, it winds up in spinal fluid. How it gets there, nobody is quite certain. Although the precise mechanics are not yet understood, nobody will deny the toxin's presence because its effects are quite acute and result in death in 70 percent of the cases.

Oster used this information for his own ends.

It happened in California in the fall of 1971 at a meeting of the International Academy of Preventive Medicine. Shortly before, in July of 1971, in Westchester County, New York, a man named Cochran died of Type A Botulism. His wife barely survived.

The cause of Cochran's death was traced to a tainted can of the Bon Vivant brand vichyssoise soup. Most newspapers carried the story. A nationwide search was launched for 6,444 cans of the product, all of which were suspected. Not all the cans were recovered, perhaps because some people kept them for souvenirs. Having a can on display in the house was fun, as long as everybody was in on the joke.

So here is Oster at the lecture, answering some of his research critics. He holds up a can of Bon Vivant vichyssoise soup to the scientists at the meeting and challenges them: "I invite you to eat some of this if you really believe large proteins are digested in the stomach!"

There were no takers.

There is little impetus to research XO. Neither the pharmaceutical manufacturers, nor the medical profession, stand to profit from a relatively simple and low-cost answer like Oster's folic acid-ascorbic acid therapy.

It would be a mistake, however, to view the situation as a conspiracy. It is, more accurately an example of benign neglect. In Oster's opinion, no profit means no interest.

Oster is not willing to accept this attitude. He has invested a remarkable amount of his time, money, and energy in a quest for answers. For him, it is an exercise in pure scientific ability. He did not embark on his research for the purpose of making himself wealthy. However, he did regain in the process a most valuable possession: his health.

And, where the big money projects have uniformly been failures, Oster's tightly disciplined little group has succeeded.

Perhaps that's why they've come under such severe fire from the establishment.

"We should have asked somebody for a million dollars," Oster says. "Then they would take us seriously."

Oster is alternately outraged and philosophical about the treatment his ideas have received.

"They throw all kinds of objections at my work," he says. "I've answered them all, if they'd only listen and do their homework," he adds pointing to his article, "Reflections on a Dietary Cause of Atherosclerosis."

"It is very disappointing to present the results of rigorous scientific research to a professional audience only to discover from the unsophistication of their criticism that they have not really read my published articles."

Oster's concern here is that all kinds of misinformation concerning his work continues to accumulate. People who hear about the XO factor from secondary sources can be totally misled.

"I do not claim," says Oster with emphasis, "that I have the one and only answer to the causes and treatment of atherosclerosis. Look at cancer. The one thing we can say about cancer is that it can be triggered by a number of causes. And, sadly there are few answers. It's the same with atherosclerosis.

"I have identified one dietary cause of the disease. I have offered an answer. I have proved the solution can work through clinical work.

"But, the debate goes on, despite the fact that more and more independent researchers around the world are now moving into this field. I welcome these new colleagues. One gets weary of carrying the fight all alone."

In a society in which the rights of the individual are considered sacred, it is the right of each person to know about biologically available BMXO. People are entitled to a choice between those foods which contain biologically available BMXO and those which do not. The public has been made aware of the hazards of smoking. They must also be told of the hazards of BMXO. Many still continue to smoke, despite the warnings; not everybody would choose to eliminate homogenized milk from their diet even if warning labels were placed on milk cartons and dairy products. Ideally dairies should create a milk free of biologically available BMXO. Until, and, if they do, they should be putting a label on their products stating:

WARNING: This food contains biologically a-vailable xanthine oxidase. Medical research has shown that xanthine oxidase may contribute to cardiovascular disease and may be hazardous to human health.

Question and Answers

Kurt A. Oster has been involved in one aspect or another of his quest to unravel one of the dietary causes of atherosclerosis for several decades. His colleague, Donald J. Ross, has worked intimately with him since 1971. Nicholas Sampsidis first started publishing material about Doctor Oster and XO for the general public in the late 1970s. Hazel Richmond Dawkins joined the effort to heighten public awareness of the XO health menace when she suggested a full-length book on the subject. As a latecomer to the scene, she was in for some surprises.

As Dawkins researched the subject and reviewed the experiments and the dramatic clinical results Oster had achieved, she came to realize she was witness to a great moment in the history of medicine. Was Oster, she wondered, a modern example of the prophet without honor? Her research showed that he was being ignored by much of the medical community. In common with other scientists who dared to tear down old ideas and to introduce new knowledge, men like Leeuwenhoek,

Pasteur, and Semmelweiss, Oster's work has been endlessly sniped at and criticized by colleagues. Even his freedom to present his solution to the public is being hampered by the FDA's curious regulations on folic acid. In their final stage of their collaboration on *The XO Factor* Dawkins presented Oster with questions on the subject.

D: If you were to venture a guess, Doctor Oster, how many researchers at universities, hospitals, and laboratories throughout the world are at present researching some aspect of XO and its connection with atherosclerosis?

O: Oh, I'd say you can count the researchers on one hand. However, it pleases me to say that these are people whose work is of the highest quality. Povoa in Brazil, Ghandi in India, Zikakis at the University of Delaware, a few others. Curiously, Zikakis may no longer be able to continue his active research. His research funding has dried up.

D: Could you estimate what percentage of the available research dollar is presently being allocated on XO versus cholesterol research?

O: Any such comparison is laughable. Over the past three decades, billions of dollars have been poured into the "popular" type of research with virtually nothing to show for it. Practically nothing has been spent on XO. Ross and I have been conducting our research at our own expense.

D: Have you any idea what percentage of the physicians in the United States have heard of XO and its connection to atherosclerosis? And of these how many fully understand the concept?

O: It's not possible to give you any accurate figures but, interestingly, quite a few have
heard of the XO concept. Very few have invested the time to read all of the work we
have published and don't fully understand the
hypothesis. I receive phone calls sporadically
from physicians from all over the country who
have been handed one of my articles or the
booklet about my work. I always write everybody back. My postage bill is substantial!

D: Does the American Medical Association hold
official views on certain areas in medicine
which you and your fellow practicing physicians must adhere to if one is to avoid being
labeled a quack?

O: The AMA doesn't hold official views per se but
it does offer guidelines in certain areas, especially concerning chronic degenerative diseases, and any physician who ignores these guidelines invites censure. Unfortunately, a professional body such as the AMA views itself as a
guardian of the status quo. The research Ross
and I are committed to naturally upsets the
status quo. So, between the establishment and
the researcher who plows into virgin territory
there is always friction.

D: Truth has a way of surfacing. Someday, Doctor
Oster, your work will become public knowledge. Perhaps this book will help. Do you feel
acceptance will come first in the United
States? Or, will it come from a country where
the ruling medical body is characterized by
more objective and innovative thinking?

O: I doubt official recognition will first come in
the United States. Based on the number of
reprint requests I receive from researchers in

certain countries, I would have to say that acceptance may first come from Japan or Europe. Swedes, Germans, and the British seem most interested in our work. Our work on XO has also raised considerable interest in some of the eastern countries, such as Czechoslovakia, Romania, and the Soviet Union.

D: Doctor Oster, you have mentioned that a person can actually get a fairly good estimate of the extent to which his or her arteries are affected by XO with the antibody test, which if you have no objections, I'll refer to as the Oster-Ross test. I think anybody who has read this book would be interested in taking this test. What must one do to have this test done?

O: Yes, the antibody test is a reliable indicator of XO related damage in the arteries. If a person's blood serum measure's more than +2 on the scale of 1 to 5, intervention with folic acid would be advisable to negate the effects of XO. Presetly we don't know how long XO remains active in the arteries. It may be a long time. The lab we use to measure XO antibody levels is here in Fairfield. Few, if any, other labs in the United States are equipped to perform the test. The test, in contrast to the therapy, could be done by mail. Any interested party can write the publisher for all the details. Since I cannot prescribe folic acid by mail, a patient would have to come to my office in Connecticut for treatment if the antibody test deemed it necessary.

D: Since folic acid is the key to your therapy program wouldn't it make life easier for you if the restrictions by the FDA were lifted?

O: Of course. The use of folic acid is freely accepted in most other countries. In Germany folic acid, is listed in the respected "rote liste" as a useful treatment for certain maladies such as psoriasis. Other researchers... Tibor Kopjak, from Indiana, has demonstrated the benefits of folic acid in microcirculation. He has obtained a United States patent for the use of folic acid as a vasodilator, so it is accepted for improving capillary circulation.

D: In what areas of your research would you like to see further work done?

O: I would like to see more autopsy work like the kind we did to determine what percentage of those who die have plasmalogen depletion in the arteries due to XO. Also it would be valuable to purify XO to a higher degree. With a pure antigen, very specific antibodies could be determined for use in diagnostic screening.

D: Perhaps the actual question I am asking is: if the cost of research was no object, and if you had all the research money you required – access to the best facilities and equipment – what studies would you conduct that might prove, beyond any doubt, that XO is the primary culprit in atherogenesis?

O: Actually, part of the beauty of our research is that it would not require the millions of dollars that have been spent on cholesterol research. However, to answer your hypothetical question, Ross and I would like to see youthful accident victims examined to establish what percentage have plasmalogen depletion in their arteries. Also, fluorescent antibody work makes it is possible to map, or trace, the sites where XO is present in arterial tissue. The procedure involves injecting highly purified BMXO into animals, such as rabbits. In response to this foreign protein, rabbits produce BMXO antibody. Once removed from the rabbits' blood this antibody is tagged with a fluorescein dye. If the BMXO-antibody-fluorescein complex is put in contact with tissue containing BMXO, it fluoresces under a fluoroscope. Diseased arterial autopsy tissue should fluoresce while healthy tissue would not. There are other experiments we could devise along this line, but in no case would it be necessary to spend $115 million of taxpayer's money as did MRFIT, *with no tangible results.*

D: You mentioned that a handful of other scientists have uncovered evidence to support your findings. Could you summarize what work these researchers have done?

O: Povoa, who flew up from Brazil to discuss our research, duplicated our work and has shown that folic acid, in addition to acting as an inhibitor of XO, may restore plasmalogen tissue in the circulatory system. Zikakis and his group at the University of Delaware have supported our research by clearly showing that XO in homogenized milk is not entirely digested in the stomach as opponents claim it is. Zikakis has shown that the strong buffering effect of milk neutralizes the acidity of gastric juice to an almost neutral pH, leaving 45 to 90 percent of ingested XO intact.

D: People often ask, "Do I have to give up milk completely?" How would you respond to this question?

O: XO can be destroyed, or denatured, by heating homogenized milk at home to a temperature of about 92° C or 195° F for about ten to fifteen seconds, which means a good simmering.

Milk drinkers will notice a difference in the taste, but this is something to which one can grow accustomed. Of course it would be infinitely preferable if the dairies stopped homogenizing milk to reduce the quantity of biologically available XO. The milk processors claim that consumers wouldn't like the taste. I'd like to point out that in the years after World War II, the dairies took several years to accustom consumers to the different taste of homogenized milk. Consumers around the world have had their milk tastes changed in the past. We're talking here of helping millions avoid serious illness. The dairy industry has the opportunity to act in the public interest. Certainly that's a point they could use to their own great advantage.

D: Which dairy products are highest in biologically available XO? Does skim milk have less XO than whole milk? Is butter safe? Does evaporated or powdered milk contain XO?

O: The type of processing a dairy product is put through determines the amount of biologically available XO in the final product. For example, butter contains no active XO. Most cheeses and yogurt, but not ice cream, do not contain XO in a biologically available form.   To best answer your question I'd like to refer you to the work done by Zikakis and Wooters who tested 195 commercially processed dairy products for XO activity. The information was published in the *Journal of Dairy Science*, June 1980. Any products which were homogenized were probably 10 to 15 percent higher in XO activity than shown on the following tables since a liposome rupturing agent to liberate XO sequestered in liposomes was not used.

Table 7 Xanthine oxidase activity in various brands of commercially processed whole milks.

Brand	Xanthine oxidase activity[a]		
	Range	$\bar{X}$	SE
A	96.2 – 156.4	126.1	16.1
B	41.4 – 68.2	59.6	5.3
C	102.1 – 148.3	126.8	12.9
D	100.4 – 170.9	138.1	17.8
D	84.9 – 139.4	113.1	10.1
E	60.7 – 98.7	78.3	6.9
F	50.9 – 74.4	62.1	5.2
F	36.2 – 58.9	48.3	5.3
G	80.5 – 129.9	104.5	11.9
H	96.5 – 174.9	139.7	18.2
A	91.7 – 152.1	121.2	14.4
I	30.9 – 48.8	36.5	4.5

[a]Enzyme activity for five purchases for each brand name product was determined polarographically in duplicates and expressed in $\mu l\ O_2$/ml per h.

Table 8 Xanthine oxidase activity in nonfat milks, skim milks, and other dairy fluids.

Product	Brand	Xanthine oxidase activity[a]		
		Range	$\bar{X}$	SE
Nonfat milk	A	14.1 – 21.8	16.0	1.3
Nonfat milk	B	20.6 – 31.0	24.4	2.9
Skim milk	D	79.8 – 119.9	105.7	12.3
Low fat (2%) milk	D	94.9 – 157.7	129.8	15.7
Low fat milk	J	86.1 – 146.1	110.7	16.0
Low fat milk	F	49.8 – 76.8	62.1	7.1
99% fat free	A	36.9 – 49.2	41.5	3.2
Skim milk	F	0 0	0	0
Low fat chocolate	C	21.3 – 34.2	27.3	3.0
Chocolate milk	F	16.5 – 26.8	20.3	2.6
Buttermilk[b]	D	0 0	0	0
Chocolate milk	H	0 0	0	0
Milk shake	K	2.6 – 5.3	4.6	.4

[a]Enzyme activity for three separate purchases for each brand name product was determined polarographically in duplicates and expressed in $\mu l\ O_2$/ml per h.

[b]Ultrapasteurized.

Table 9 Xanthine oxidase activity in commercially processed powdered milk, evaporated milk, and butter.

Product	Brand	Xanthine oxidase activity[a]		
		Range	$\bar{X}$	SE
Evaporated milk	D	0	0	...
Evaporated milk	L	0	0	...
Evaporated milk	M	0	0	...
Evaporated milk	N	0	0	...
Evaporated skim milk	N	0	0	...
Instant dry milk	N	0	0	...
Evaporated milk	I	0	0	...
Instant dry milk	D	113.6 – 146.3	126.5	6.9
Evaporated milk	A	0	0	...
Instant dry milk	O	0	0	...
Instant milk	P	0	0	...
Infant formula	Q	0	0	...
Infant formula	R	15.4 – 24.4	20.1	2.0
Butter	S	28.4 – 39.4	32.5	2.8
Butter	T	0	0	...
Butter	U	0	0	...
Butter	O	0	0	...
Butter	V	0	0	...
Butter	W	0	0	...
Butter	B	0	0	...
Butter	X	0	0	...

[a]Enzyme activity for two separate purchases for each brand name product was determined polarographically in duplicates and expressed in $\mu l\ O_2$/g per h.

Table 10   Xanthine oxidase activity in yogurts and ice creams.

Product	Brand	Xanthine oxidase activity[a]		
		Range	$\bar{X}$	SE
Yogurt	Y	0	0	0
Yogurt	Z	0	0	0
Yogurt	J	1.9 – 3.1	2.2	.1
Yogurt	S	0	0	0
Vanilla ice cream	a	1.8 – 2.9	2.1	.1
Vanilla ice cream	b	6.9 – 10.9	9.6	.5
Vanilla ice cream	F	0	0	0
Vanilla ice cream	C	0	0	0
Vanilla ice cream	d	32.4 – 49.3	40.3	3.7
Vanilla ice cream	F	0	0	0
Vanilla ice cream	e	29.8 – 44.8	34.7	3.4
Vanilla ice cream	f	22.0 – 34.2	27.2	2.9
Vanilla ice cream	J	0	0	0
Vanilla ice cream	C	0	0	0

[a]Enzyme activity for three separate purchases for each brand name product was determined polarographically in duplicates and expressed in $\mu l\ O_2$/g per h.

Journal of Dairy Science Vol. 63, No. 6, 1980

Table 11   Xanthine oxidase activity in commercially processed cream.

Product	Brand	Xanthine oxidase activity[a]		
		Range	$\bar{X}$	SE
Ultra-pasteurized light cream	C	0	0	0
Ultra-pasteurized heavy cream	C	0	0	0
Light cream	D	63.9 – 96.1	78.5	7.0
Heavy cream[b]	D	341.3 – 473.0	404.9	38.2
Half N Half	D	72.6 – 104.9	88.1	7.1
Ultra-pasteurized light cream	A	0	0	0
Ultra-pasteurized heavy cream	A	0	0	0
Half N Half[b]	A	290.2 – 407.4	344.4	30.2
Half N Half[b]	C	187.4 – 271.2	227.5	19.8
Sterilized whipping cream	D	0	0	0
Sour cream	S	6.2 – 9.6	8.7	.5
Sour cream	F	7.4 – 10.1	9.2	.6
Sour cream	A	0	0	0
Sour Half N Half cream	S	9.0 – 14.9	11.5	1.0
Half N Half	B	21.9 – 32.7	27.8	2.4
Light cream	j	0	0	0
Whipping cream	j	0	0	0
Whipping cream	I	0	0	0
Ultra-pasteurized light cream	I	3.0 – 4.9	4.3	.3
Ultra-pasteurized whipping cream	A	3.0 – 4.9	4.4	.3
Cream topping	D	0	0	0
Whipping cream	h	0	0	0
Cream topping	i	0	0	0
Ultra-pasteurized whipping cream	A	3.2 – 5.4	4.4	.4

[a]Enzyme activity for four separate purchases for each brand name product was determined in duplicate or triplicate samples polarographically and expressed in $\mu l\ O_2$/ml per h.

[b]Enzyme activity is based on four separate purchases of triplicate samples.

Journal of Dairy Science Vol. 63, No. 6, 1980

Table 12 Xanthine oxidase activity in domestic and imported cheeses.

Variety	Xanthine oxidase activity[a]		
	Range	X̄	SE
St. Benoit	381.2 – 452.0	420.4	20.0
99% Fat free Cottage[b]	269.4 – 379.9	349.2	29.3
Cottage[b]	252.3 – 350.1	310.1	27.7
Monterey Jack	278.9 – 344.4	303.9	14.6
Butter Nip	233.4 – 287.3	269.2	12.9
May-Bud Natural Muenster	229.4 – 278.4	251.2	10.9
Double Gloucester	201.3 – 256.3	237.7	9.9
Sharp Cheddar	217.5 – 260.6	236.8	8.6
Non-fat Cottage[b]	181.3 – 269.9	227.8	21.3
Longhorn Cheddar	201.4 – 244.1	227.7	11.4
Cutter	199.9 – 250.4	227.7	10.9
Cottage[b]	176.4 – 249.1	216.4	16.2
Cottage[b]	183.8 – 248.1	216.4	15.1
Smoked Edam Hickory Natural	166.2 – 221.6	206.7	9.1
Swiss	186.5 – 230.8	204.2	8.8
Gouda	160.1 – 198.9	188.6	6.7
Stella Provolone[b]	141.1 – 209.6	178.3	13.9
Old Fashion Cheddar (sharp)	158.0 – 181.0	173.2	4.9
Extra Sharp Cheddar	142.0 – 180.4	168.4	5.4
Swiss	152.6 – 180.8	168.3	4.8
Extra Sharp Cheddar	128.9 – 181.0	159.7	7.3
Valio Gruyere	133.4 – 174.0	154.5	6.4
New York Style Cheddar	129.1 – 158.9	148.4	6.3
Cottage[b]	119.9 – 170.4	140.4	9.6
Wensleydale	123.8 – 152.0	137.2	6.3
Cottage[b]	120.4 – 167.8	132.3	9.3
Brie	115.4 – 141.9	125.9	4.7
Clearfield Swiss	107.3 – 140.1	118.5	5.1
Caerphilly	99.9 – 121.4	113.1	4.9
Mild Cheddar	87.8 – 119.0	106.9	4.7
St. Ohio	91.4 – 110.0	104.2	3.2
Provolone	87.3 – 113.4	102.3	4.0
Cracker Barrel Mild White Cheddar	89.7 – 116.1	101.9	4.9
Appenzeller	84.2 – 118.7	95.6	4.7
Mohawk Valley Limberger	86.9 – 109.6	91.3	4.1
New York Cheddar	77.4 – 100.4	89.6	4.1
Provolone	76.4 – 93.2	89.3	3.9
Master Quality Provolone	60.1 – 72.0	65.9	2.9
Clearfield Provolone	59.2 – 70.3	62.4	2.8
Bella Dolca	49.8 – 63.9	58.5	2.9
Kasseri	49.6 – 61.3	58.3	2.0
May-Bud Gouda	53.0 – 64.1	57.2	2.2
Canadian Cheddar	49.4 – 60.9	55.0	2.1
Mozzarella[b]	39.8 – 68.5	50.6	4.6
Jailsbury	38.4 – 48.9	47.8	2.0
Emmnthaler	38.3 – 47.0	42.7	1.8
Cracker Barrel Mellow White Cheddar	29.9 – 37.8	32.1	1.2
Cottage[b]	23.9 – 35.0	30.7	2.2
Liederkranz[b]	23.6 – 32.9	27.9	2.0
Swedish Ambrosia	24.2 – 29.0	25.8	1.1
American	23.4 – 28.4	25.2	1.0
Cracker Barrel Sharp Cheddar[b]	21.5 – 27.2	24.3	.9
Brandy Cheddar[b]	18.9 – 27.3	23.5	1.1
Sharp	16.4 – 23.6	20.0	.9
Hernsgaurd	14.9 – 20.9	18.7	.8
Leyeden	15.4 – 20.2	17.8	.8
Graddost	15.4 – 20.2	17.8	.8
Ricotta[b]	14.6 – 21.2	17.6	1.2
Citation	14.2 – 19.4	17.6	.8
Romano	15.0 – 19.1	17.6	.7
Cheddar Processed Cheese Spread	12.1 – 16.4	14.4	.5
American	12.4 – 17.6	13.6	.6
Dutch Edam	10.9 – 16.4	13.5	.6
Estrom	11.1 – 15.9	13.5	.5
Danish Fontina	11.4 – 15.0	13.5	.4
Mild Longhorn Colby	10.9 – 14.9	12.5	.4
May-Bud Blue	7.9 – 12.0	9.1	.4
Cracker Barrel Sharp White Cheddar	5.7 – 10.4	8.8	.4
Cheese Spread	3.8 – 5.0	4.5	.1
Camembert Soft Ripened	1.0 – 1.5	1.2	0
Cottage[b]	0	0	0
Cottage[b]	0	0	0
Cream[b]	0	0	0

Table 12   (continued) Xanthine oxidase activity in domestic and imported cheeses.

Variety	Xanthine oxidase activity[a]		
	Range	X̄	SE
Cream[b]	0	0	0
Cream[b]	0	0	0
Cream[b]	0	0	0
American Processed Cheese Spread	0	0	0
Rondele Soft Ripen	0	0	0
Cheese Wiz	0	0	0
Treasure Cave Blue	0	0	0
Sharp Old English	0	0	0
American	0	0	0
Clearfield American	0	0	0
Clearfield Sharp	0	0	0
Mozzarella[b]	0	0	0
American	0	0	0
Smoked Flavored Cheese Spread	0	0	0
Havarti	0	0	0
Tilsiter	0	0	0
Lappi	0	0	0
Greek Feta[b]	0	0	0
Gouda[b]	0	0	0
Tybo	0	0	0
Danish Cream	0	0	0
Gourmandise	0	0	0
Bianco	0	0	0
Port Salut	0	0	0
Provolone	0	0	0
Swedish Tilsiter	0	0	0
Noekkelost	0	0	0
Farm	0	0	0
Jolli Noix	0	0	0
Koppelzak	0	0	0
Blue	0	0	0
Plain	0	0	0
Sharp	0	0	0
Mild Brick	0	0	0
Samsoe	0	0	0
Bon Jolli	0	0	0
Italian Provolone[b]	0	0	0
Grated Parmesan[b]	0	0	0

[a]Enzyme activity for one or two separate purchases for each product was determined polarographically in duplicates and expressed in μl O_2/g per h.

[b]Enzyme activity is based on two purchases of duplicate samples.

D: What direction is your research taking right now?

O: My primary efforts lie in treating patients with folic acid. Ross and I could spend the rest of our lives performing additional experiments to prove our findings, and certain people would still refuse to accept them. I know of some colleagues who cling to the cholesterol idea even after they've had a heart attack. Ross and I have convinced ourselves beyond a shadow of a doubt that XO is a chief threat to health and we believe we have found how to retard the progress of atherosclerosis. I will spend my time constructively, lecturing and helping those who come to me for therapy.

D: The physician William Kelly, once observed in his book *One Answer to Cancer*, that when one looked at the history of diseases such as polio, tuberculosis, rickets, diabetes, as well as several of the infectious diseases, one finds an interesting pattern.

First a disease appears to be many different diseases, depending on which organ or part of the body is attacked (heart attack, stroke, poor leg circulation, etc.).

Second the disease seems to be caused by many different things.

Third eventually someone discovers that many of the different diseases are in truth one disease.

Fourth someone else figures out that since there is only one disease, there must be one cause.

Fifth everyone thinks he has found the cause.

Sixth there is a long period of trial and error where everything from snake oil to cobalt is the "cure."

Seventh someone really finds the simple solution, ususally on his own, independent of institutional or government grants and controls.

Eighth this individual spends the rest of his or her life "crying in the wilderness," trying to get organized medicine to use the ideas or cure. But because it is so simple, organized medicine ignores the work and refuses even to consider it until...

Ninth a promoter, often a large drug company, sees an opportunity to make a large fortune.

Tenth the drug company then runs a small study of say 28 or 74 cases, and announces a great discovery.

Eleventh the drug company rushes many salesmen with free samples to the doctors' offices.

Twelfth the innovative researcher becomes "accepted," although often dead by this time; the drug company is wealthy.

Does this pattern apply to your case?

O: Very much so, except the diseases of the arteries are complex and have more than one cause.   Also, as of yet, the drug companies haven't spotted the profit potential in the folic acid–ascorbic acid formula. If the drug companies had adequate patent protection, there could be a substantial profit in marketing the formulation. Consider all the people who could benefit from it. Sooner or later, this historical trend you've just described will be fulfilled. Then perhaps we'll see a reduction of much of the atherosclerosis that plagues the world.

Notes

CHAPTER 1

Laying the Foundation

Frederickson, D. S., Levy, R. I., Lees, R. S., *New England J. Medicine*, "Fat Transport in Lipoproteins — An Integrated Approach to Mechanisms and Disorders," 1967. 276:34-44.

A Hypothesis is Created

Oster, K. A., Hope-Ross, P., "Plasmal Reaction in a Case of Recent Myocardial Infarction," *American J. Cardiology*, 1966. 17:83-85.

CHAPTER 2

Atherogenesis — Another Perspective On How The Disease Starts

DeBakey, M., Gotto, A., *The Living Heart*, New York: McKay. 1977.

Oster, K. A., "Plasmalogen Disease: A New Concept of the Etiology of the Atherosclerotic Process, *Amer. J. Clinical Research*, April 1971, Vol. 2, No. 1. pp. 30-35, April 1971.

Questions in Search of Solutions

Morgan, E. J., *Biochemistry Journal*, 1926. 161:1280.

Oster, K. A., Mulinos, M. G., "Tissue Aldehydes and Their Reaction With Amines," *J. Pharma. Exp. Thera.*, 1944. 80:132.

Oster, K. A., "Treatment of Angina Pectoris According to a New Theory of Its Origins," *Cardiology Digest*, 1968. 3:29-34.

Altman, J. K., *New York Times*, September 22, 1981.

Ross, D. J., Ptaszynski, M., Oster, K. A., "The Presence of Ectopic Xanthine Oxidase in Atherosclerotic Plaques and Myocardial Tissues," *Proc. Soc. Exp. Biol. Med.*, 1973. 144:523-526.

Around the World in Search of Facts

World Health Statistics Annual, World Health, Aug.-Sept. p. 11, 1970.

Butz, W. T., *How Americans Use Their Dairy Foods*, National Dairy Council, Chicago, Ill. p. 15, 1971.

Is Milk a Natural?

Ross, D. J., Sharnick, S. V., Oster, K. A., "Liposomes as a Proposed Vehicle for the Persorption of Bovine Xanthine Oxidase," *Proc. Soc. Exp. Biol. Med.*, 163:141-145. 1981.

Full Circle

Oster, K. A., Oster, J., Ross, D. J., "Immune Response to Bovine Xanthine Oxidase in Atherosclerotic Patients," *American Laboratory*, August 1974. 41-47.

Rzucidlo, S. J., Zikakis, J. P., *Proc. Soc. Exp. Biol. Med.*, 1979. 160:477-482.

CHAPTER 3

Plasmalogen Disease Therapy

Kalckar, H. M., Klenow, H., *J. Biol. Chem.*, 1948. 172:349-350.

Scientific Papers

Oster, K. A., "The Absorption and Inhibition of Xanthine Oxidase," *American Laboratory*, October 1976.

CHAPTER 4

A Disease of the Young

Enos, W. F., Holmes, R. H., Beyer, J., "Coronary Disease Among United States Soldiers Killed in Action in Korea. *JAMA*, 1953. 152:1090-1093.

Jaffe, D., Hartroft, W. S., Manning, M., Eleta, G., "Coronary Arteries in Newborn Children: Intimal Variations in Longitudinal Sections and Their Relationship to Clinical and Experimental Data," *Acta Paediat.*, Scand. Supple., 219, 1971.

The Many Faces of Atherosclerosis

Arthur, Fisher, *The Healthy Heart*, Time-Life Books, 1981. p. 58.

DeBakey, Michael, Gotto, Antonio, *The Living Heart*, New York: David McKay Co., 1977, pp. ix, x.

Proliferation of an Ancient Disease

Ruffer, M. A., "On Arterial Lesions Found in Egyptian Mummies (1580 BC-525 AD), *J. Path. Bacteriol.*, Cambridge, 1910, XV:453-462.

Keys, A. "Coronary Heart Disease – The Global Picture." *Atherosclerosis*, 22:149-192, 1975.

Keys, A., Kimura, N., Kusukawa, A., Bronte-Stewart, B., Larsen, N. P., Keys, M. H., "Lessons From Serum Cholesterol Studies in Japan, Hawaii, and Los Angeles," *Ann. Intern. Med.*, 48:83-94, 1958.

Vlodaver, Z., Kahn, H. A., Neufeld, H. N., "The Coronary Arteries in Early Life in Three Different Ethnic Groups," *Circulation*, 39:541-550, 1969.

Rabinowitch, I. M., "Clinical and Other Observations on Canadian Eskimos in the Eastern Artic," *Canadian Med. Assn. J.*, 34:487-501, 1936.

Treating the Symptoms

Friedan, Betty, "Twenty Years After the Feminine Mystique," *The New York Times Magazine*, February 1983.

Physician's Management, "Is Preventive Medicine Really Possible?" July 1981, pp. 52-61.

A Dietary Cause

Roussos, G. G., *Biochim. Biophys. Acta.*, 1963. pp. 73-338.

The Elusive Causes

Gruberg, E. R., Raymond, S. A., *Beyond Cholesterol, Vitamin B6, Arteriosclerosis, and Your Heart*, New York: St. Martin's Press, 1981.

Van Buchem, F. S. P., "Atherosclerosis and Nutrition," *Nutr. Dieta*, 4:122-147, 1962.

Biskind, M. S., "The Technic of Nutritional Therapy," *Amer. Jour. Dig. Dis.* September 26, 1952, pp. 57ff.

Oates, J. A., "The 1983 Nobel Prize in Physiology and Medicine," *Science*, November 19, 1982, 218:765ff.

CHAPTER 5

Madison Avenue Medicine

Consumer Reports, "What Everyone Knows About Diet and Heart Disease May Not Be True." May 1981.

Pinckney, E. R., Pinckney, C., *The Cholesterol Controversy*, Sherbourne Press, Los Angeles, 1973.

Antar, M. A., Ohlson, M. A., Hodges, R. E., "Changes in Retail Market Food Supplies an the United States in the Last Seventy Years in Relation to the Incidence of Coronary Heart Disease, With Special Reference to Dietary Carbohydrates and Essential Fatty Acids," *American J. Clinical Nutr.*, Vol. 14, March 1964. pp. 169-178.

Suspect the Statistics

Rothman, K. J., "The Rise and Fall of Epidemiology," *New England J. Med.*, March 5, 1981, 10:600-602.

How Human is a Rabbit?

Ignatovski, A. I., "Influence de la Nourriture Animale sur L'Organisme des Lapins," *Arch. Med. Exo.*, 20:1-20, 1908.

Anitschkow, N., Chalatow, S., "Ueber Experimentalle Cholesterinsteatose und Bedeutung fur die Entstehung Einiger Pathologisher Prozesse," *Centralbl. f. Allg. Path. u. Path. Anat.*, 24:1, 1913

Special Interest Groups

Solomon, H. A., "Can Coronary Heart Disease Be Altered or Prevented Through Modification of Associated Risk Factors?" *Cardiology Counterpoint* July 1981. CPC Communications, Greenwich, Ct. This article comprises a debate between Dr. George V. Mann and Dr. P. Herbert.

The Cholesterol Fallacy Exposed
Six Straight Answers

Peterson, J. E., *Circulation*, August 1960, 22:247

Psychosomatic Medicine, September/October 1971. 33:399. Two U.S. Navy Experiments.

Elek, S. R., "Stress and Physiology," *Bulletin of the Beverly Hills District of the Los Angeles County Medical Association*, September 1972, quoting Friedman, M., et al., "Changes in the Serum Cholesterol and Blood Clotting Time in Men Subject to Cyclic Variation of Occupational Stress," *Circulation*, 17:852, May 1958.

Tract, Myron, Professor of Pathology at Columbia University College of Physicians and Surgeons has compiled a list of commonly used drugs that will cause false results when blood cholesterol is measured (*Consultant*, September, 1972). Twenty-six of the 49 drugs studied altered the cholesterol level sufficiently to yield an error in the test results.

Various hormones, whether produced naturally by the body or taken as medicines, will severly alter one's blood cholesterol without causing heart disease. If one takes any cortisone product – and there are over 100 different variations of this steroid drug – blood cholesterol will go up. (*Medical World News*, August 6, 1971.) An increase in the amount of insulin in the body will also cause a concurrent elevated blood cholesterol (*Medical Tribune*, June 16, 1971; *Cardiology Abstracts*, September 1968.

Friedman, Meyer, described "neurogenic hypercholesterolemia," and the relationship of the occupational stress to elevated serum cholesterol in *Circulation*, 22:852, May 1958, and *Circulation*, 29:874, June 1964.

For a reference to how our bodies have the ability to stabilize our blood cholesterol no matter what one eats, see *Annals of the New York Academy of Sciences*, 149:838. November 21, 1968. Also, "Cholesterol Absorption vs. Cholesterol Synthesis in Man," *Nutrition Reviews*, 28: 11, January 1970.

The list of scientific material published on the damage caused by eating an excess of polyunsaturated fats is extensive. Pinckney, E., *The Cholesterol Controversy*, Sherbourne Press, Los Angeles, 1973, has a lengthy list in the Annotated Bibliography, pp. 127-131. A brief sampling of such papers follows: Mead, James, F., "Dietary Polyunsaturated Fatty Acids as Potential Toxic Factors," *Chemtech*, American Chemical Society, p. 70, February 1972; details of toxicity of corn oil, including death, *The Journal of Clinical Pharmacology*, p. 137, May/June 1969; "Nutrition in Relation to Cancer," *Nutrition Today*, January 1972; for a detailed explanation of how polyunsaturates actually can cause cancer, see the *American Journal of Medicine*, 35:143, August 1963; *Medical Tribune*, September 29, 1971.

Oster, K. A., "The Cholesterol Bias Revisited, A Different Approach to a Dietary Cause of Atherosclerosis," *Journal of the International Academy of Preventive Medicine*, VIII:1, 43-46, Winter 1983.

For a comprhensive list of the many worldwide studies that contradict the idea that a diet high in saturated fats contributes to heart disease, see the classic critical review of 98 different reports which show *no* definitive relationship (*American Journal of Public Health*, 60:1477, August 1970). Dr. George Mann's many studies of the Masai (*Journal of Atherosclerosis Research*, 4:289, 1964); others have confirmed Dr. Mann's information: Dr. K. Biss, *The New England Journal of Medicine*, April 1, 1971, and *Pathology and Microbiology*, 35:198, 1970. A study of Alaskan Eskimos who eat a diet high in saturated fats and cholesterol but have an almost total absence of heart disease (*Fat Consumption and Coronary Disease*, New York: Philosophical Library, 1958).

CHAPTER 6

The Milky Way

Robbins, William, *The American Food Scandal*, pp. 205, 206, 209, New York: William Morrow & Co., 1974.

Ross, D. J., Sharnick, S. V., Oster, K. A., "Liposomes as a Proposed Vehicle for the Persorption of Bovine Xanthine Oxidase," *Proc. Soc. Exper. Biol. Med.*, 163, 141-145, 1980.

Experts Clash on Nutrition Policy

Eliott, J., "Experts Clash on Nutrition Policy," Medical News, *JAMA*, December 14, 1979, 242:24, 2645-2653.

Myth of the Healthy Savage

Moncema, T., AMA Department of Food and Nutrition, Chicago, letter in *JAMA*'s "Questions and Answers," January 4, 1980, Vol. 243, No. 1.

Glory of the Long Distance Runner

The American Medical Joggers Association Newsletter, July 1981.

Cerqueira, M. T., McMurry Fry, M., Connor, W. E., "The Food and Nutrient Intakes of the Tarahumara Indians of

Mexico," *The American Journal of Clinical Nutrition,* April 1979, pp. 905-915.

Pennington, C. W., *The Tarahumar of Mexico,* University of Utah Press, Salt Lake City, Utah, 1963.

More Myths: The Masai of East Africa

World Health Statistics Annual, World Health, Aug-Sept. 1970, p. 11.

Butz, W. T., "How Americans Use Their Dairy Foods," National Dairy Council, Chicago, p. 15, 1970.

Early Warning Signals

Feldschuh, J., Gambino, R., "Extreme Central Acidosis from Abbott Epinephrine," *American Journal of Medicine,* January 1983, Vol. 74, 30-32.

Dorfman, Dan, "Heart Drug Stirs Trouble for Maker Abbott and the FDA," New York *News,* February 9, 1983

FDA Commissioner Uneasy About Business Integrity

New York Times, April 7, 1966 "Excerpts from Dr. Goddard's Address."

The High and Mighty Tainted

Broad, W. J., "U.S. to Penalize Heart Researcher on Fraudulent Project at Harvard," *New York Times,* February 16, 1983, pp. 1, A23.

Hunt, M., "A Fraud That Shook the World of Science," *New York Times Magazine,* November 1, 1981, pp. 42-75.

Broad, W. J., "Fraud in Science Taints the High and Mighty," *New York Times,* March 20, 1983, p. 20E.

Knox, R., "The Harvard Fraud Case: Where Does the Problem Lie?" *JAMA,* April 8, 1983, 249, No. 14, pp. 1797-1807.

Riddled With Doubt

Knox, R., "The Harvard Fraud Case: Where Does the Problem Lie?" *JAMA*, April 8, 1983, 249, No. 14, p. 1806.

Broad, W. J., "Fraud in Science Taints the High and Mighty," *New York Times*, March 20, 1983, p. 20E.

Broad, W. J., Wade, N., "Science's Faulty Fraud Detectors," *Psychology Today*, November 1982, pp. 51-55.

Hixon, J., *The Patchwork Mouse*, Anchor Press, Doubleday, New York, 1976.

"Books in Review," *American Medical News*, April 5, 1976.

Which Institution Has Status?

Zikakis, J., Treece, J. M., *Journal of Dairy Science*, 1970. Vol. 53, 644ff.

Pavoa, H., et al, *Acta. Biol. Med. Germ.*, 1973. Band 31, Seite 897-898.

Schloss, O. M., "The Intestinal Absorption of Antigenic Protein," Harvey Lectures, Ser. 20:156-187, 1924-25.

Isselbacher, K., Warsaw, A., Walker, A., *Gasteroenterology*, 1974. Vol. 66: 987-992.

Davies, D. F., Davies, J. R., Richard, M. A., *Jour. of Atherosclerosis Research*, 1969, Vol. 9, 103-107.

Davies, D. F., et al, *Lancet*, 1974, pp. 1012-1014.

Greenbank, G. R., Pallansch, M., *Jour. of Dairy Science*, 1962. Vol. 45, 958ff.

Room for Rebuttal

Oster, K. A., "Reflections on a Dietary Cause of Atherosclerosis," *Biologisk Medicin, The Swedish Journal of Biological Medicine*, September 1983, No. 3.

Gregoriadis, G., *New England J. Med.*, 1976, 295:704.

Deeths, H. C., "Homogenized Milk and Atherosclerotic Disease — A Review," *J. Dairy Science*, Vol. 66, 1419-1435, July 1983

Al-Khalidi, U. A. S., Chaglassian, T. H., "The Species Distribution of Xanthine Oxidase," *Am. J. Dig. Di.*, 1973. 18:15-22.

CHAPTER 7

Questions and Answers

Zikakis, J. P., Wooters, S. C., "Activity of Xanthine Oxidase in Dairy Products," *J. Dairy Science*, Vol. 63, 6:893-904, June 1980.

Original Article

Treatment of Angina Pectoris According to a New Theory of Its Origin

KURT A. OSTER, M.D.,* *Bridgeport, Connecticut*

In a recent case of fatal myocardial infarction a selective disappearance of plasmalogen from heart muscle cells was noted.[1] This observation, together with prior studies on the distribution and the physiologic behavior of plasmalogens, has led to a new theory of a possible cause of myocardial infarction and angina pectoris.

Plasmalogen, discovered in 1924[2] was first considered to be an acetal phosphatide.[3] Later it was found that an unsaturated fatty acid is also a constituent of plasmalogen, and the following formulation is now generally accepted:

$$CH_2\!-\!O\!-\!CH = CH\!-\!R_1$$
$$CH\!-\!O\!-\!CO\!-\!R_2$$
$$CH_2\!-\!O\!-\!P\!\!\stackrel{\displaystyle O}{=}\!\!O$$
$$O\!-\!CH_2\!-\!CH_2\!-\!N^+(CH_3)_3$$

R_1=fatty aldehyde residue
R_2=unsaturated fatty acid residue

Investigators[4] demonstrated that choline plasmalogen is prevalent in heart muscle but is found in only small amounts in the brain and may act as a substrate for phospholipase A (lecithinase A) which is known to hydrolyze lecithin.[5]

Plasmalogen and a phospholipase A-like enzyme are usually present in normal heart muscle. The enzyme

1. Oster, K. A., & Hope-Ross, P., *Amer. J. Cardiol.*, 17:83-85,1966.
2. Feulgen, R., & Voit, K., *Pfluegers Arch. Ges. Physiol.*, 206:389-410,1924.
3. Feulgen, R., & Bersin, T., *Z. Physiol. Chem.*, 260:217-245,1939.
*Chairman of the Department of Medicine, Park City Hospital.

4. Klenk, E., & Gehrmann, G., *Hoppe Seyler Z. Physiol. Chem.*, 292:110-117,1953.
5. Rapport, M. M., & Franzl, R. E., *J. Biol. Chem.*, 225:851-857,1957.

may be activated by calcium or by catecholamines, effecting a hydrolysis of plasmalogen, resulting in the formation, as split products, of plasmal plus a combined form of glycerophosphorocholine with an unsaturated fatty acid. In normal hearts this process would be continuous and reversible. Considering the cited disappearance of plasmalogen from heart muscle, it may be concluded that if hydrolysis becomes unbalanced by an excess of enzyme activity, plasmalogen would then disappear from the affected area and subsequent cell death, or infarction, would result. In angina pectoris the hydrolytic process is quantitatively lesser, resulting in a probable diminution rather than in a disappearance of plasmalogens. Free phospholipase A, deprived of its substrate, is a powerful algesic and could be a cause of the severe pain experienced in angina pectoris and myocardial infarction.[6]

Experimental proof of the foregoing theory is inherently difficult, since the site of the chemopathologic processes is the heart muscle cell. These processes are herewith offered as a possible explanation for those cases of myocardial infarction (approximately one third of the known total) for which none of the commonly accepted reasons for infarction, such as severe coronary atherosclerosis or coronary thrombosis, can be found despite thorough tissue investigation. Admittedly, animal experiments do not always simulate human pathology and may, furthermore, lead to therapeutic attempts at correction of the yardstick of the disease rather than the disease itself, a substitution now encountered in the current efforts to depress serum cholesterol levels.[7] To prove the author's plasmalogen theory with special emphasis on its postulated reversible form in angina pectoris, attempts were made to restore the depleted plasmalogens to the heart muscle. If such a plasmalogen restoration could be accomplished by the use of drugs with no known vasodilating, reoxygenating, or lactic acid-neutralizing action, thus ruling out prevailing theories of drug therapy, it should be considered meaningful in support of the plasmalogen-based theory.

Prolonged observation of plasmalogen distribution in animals and humans has made the author acutely aware of three distinct distribution qualities of these compounds: (1) their selective appearance in only some of the same functional units within an organ, e.g., kidney; (2) their response in distribution in certain anatomic positions to the influence of male and female hormones; and (3) their almost complete absence from normal liver cells.[8] This last observation was made the fulcrum of the new approach to angina pectoris therapy. It had been demonstrated that xanthine oxidase, normally present in the liver, was capable of oxidizing plasmal and thereby contributing to the oxidation of plasmalogens and their absence of histochemical demonstrability in normal liver tissue.[9] It was presumed that prevent-

6. Meldrum, B. S., Pharmacol. Rev., 17:393-445, 1965.

7. Yerushalmy, J., Controversy in Internal Medicine, W. B. Saunders, Philadelphia, 1966. P. 659-668.
8. Oster, K. A., Endocrinology, 36:92-97,1945.
9. Oster, K. A., & Mulinos, M. G., J. Pharmacol. Exp. Ther., 80:132-138,1944.

ing xanthine oxidase from oxidizing plasmalogen would increase the concentration of these substances in the blood and would effect their restoration to the depleted areas in the heart muscle in cases of angina pectoris. Creation of such a liver-heart axis should then lead to a diminution of angina pectoris attacks, especially those unrelated to effort, emotion, or food intake, the so-called decubital or nocturnal angina.

Since the theory demands that an appreciable quantity of plasmalogen leave the liver in its unoxidized state, the influence of any drug designed to bring about this effect must depend, of necessity, on dosage-response. There must be sufficient blockage of enzyme action in the liver to produce enough plasmalogen for effective restoration to the depleted areas of the heart.

The ability to inhibit xanthine oxidase demonstrated by the drug allopurinol* has led to its recent introduction to the medical armamentarium specifically for the prevention and treatment of gout. Although it has been claimed that allopurinol does not inhibit the oxidation of smaller aldehyde molecules, it was deemed worthwhile to titrate the action of this drug, which has no known effect on the vascular system and the heart, on patients suffering from angina pectoris.

The response of angina pectoris to drugs is notoriously unpredictable. However, to date, four patients, three women and one man, have been treated with allopurinol with amazing success. The need of these patients for nitroglycerine was defi-

*Zyloprim®, Burroughs Wellcome, Tuckahoe, New York.

nitely diminished. The drug was given in increasing amounts to rule out placebo effects. With a 200 mg. dosage (two, 100 mg. tablets daily) there was no change reported in either the frequency or severity of the attacks. Essentially the same lack of response was obtained when the dose was increased to 400 mg. daily (four, 100 mg. tablets). However, after the introduction of a daily 600 mg. dosage, two tablets of 100 mg. three times a day, all patients reported an unquestionable diminution of the angina pectoris attacks, both as to severity and frequency.

Case Reports

CASE 1

A woman aged 58, had experienced for about one year daily attacks of angina pectoris at approximately 5:30 a.m., which were relieved three to four minutes after sublingual application of nitroglycerine. Since she usually experienced some additional chest pain during the day, her average nitroglycerine intake was eight to ten tablets daily. The angina attacks were not curtailed by short-acting coronary vasodilators nor by the long-acting modifications. For many years this patient had a hypercholesterolemia ranging from 330 to 430 mg. per cent. Her weight and blood pressure were normal.

On January 30, 1967, the patient was instructed to take one-100 mg. allopurinol tablet twice daily. On February 24, after 3 and one-half weeks on this dosage she reported no relief from her angina pectoris attacks. At that time the dosage was increased to 100 mg. allopurinol four times a day. Two weeks later, on March 10, she stated that there was no appreciable change in her chest pain. She had experienced, however, some nocturia as a new symptom. Allopurinol was now increased to two tablets of 100 mg. three times daily, a total dose of 600 mg. each day. Until this time the patient had been taking erithryltetranitrate four times a day. This medication was now discontinued. On March 20 after 10 days on the 600 mg. dosage, she claimed that for the first time her attacks were of greatly diminished severity. though still as frequent as previously. By March 24 the attacks were definitely of lessened severity.

Her serum cholesterol at this time was 340 mg. per cent.

On April 7, still on 600 mg. allopurinol daily, she stated that she required but two to three nitroglycerine tablets a day, in contrast to her previous daily consumption of eight to 10 tablets. The patient was still awakened by chest pain in the early morning, but she described the pain as being so short-lived that it subsided almost before she could reach the nitroglycerine tablets on her night table, happily comparing this situation with the previous three to four minute interval of pain between administration of nitroglycerine and the onset of relief. She also reported the ability to continue normal activity even when taking nitroglycerine during the day. In the past she had found it necessary to sit down and wait until the attack of pain had subsided.

This patient continued on allopurinol 600 mg. daily with the same relief of symptoms. When a reduction of the dose to 400 mg. a day was tried, the angina pectoris again became so severe that the patient herself, on the fourth day of the reduced medication, resumed the 600 mg. daily regimen, with relief of her symptoms. Incidentally, her serum cholesterol rose to over 400 mg. per cent during this period with no evident aggravation of her symptoms. A double-blind study of the administration of the drug produced an alarming recurrence of severe angina pectoris pain lasting for about 20 minutes and responding poorly to nitroglycerine. This occurred during a period of placebo medication.

CASE 2

A woman of 68 had suffered for many years with auricular fibrillation and had experienced several attacks of pulmonary edema. Therapy included quinidine, digitalis, and diuretics. In April, 1967, she was hospitalized with acute pulmonary edema which was successfully treated. However, the patient experienced severe attacks of morning angina pectoris for which sublingual nitroglycerine was required. When she was given allopurinol 100 mg. four times a day there was no change in her condition. However, with administration of two, 100 mg. tablets three times daily (600 mg. total) the angina pectoris did not recur. Following release from the hospital this patient was instructed to reduce her daily allopurinol intake to 400 mg. with resultant prompt recurrence of morning angina pectoris. Once more, increasing the daily dosage to 600 mg. caused relief of her painful attacks. Her usual serum cholesterol concentration of approximately 300 mg. per cent remained unchanged by the administration of allopurinol.

CASE 3

A man aged 65 experienced angina pectoris with mild exertion and sometimes even when at rest. His weight was normal, blood pressure 140/80, and pulse rate 76 with regular rhythm. As of October, 1966, his nitroglycerine requirement was 40 to 60 tablets per week. His serum cholesterol level was 170 mg. per cent and the ECG showed a 1° AV block. Placing him on isosorbide dinitrate therapy resulted in a reduction of his nitroglycerine intake to about 10 to 12 tablets per week. Nevertheless, the patient still complained of substernal "burning," which was ascribed to a hiatus hernia. On April 24, 1967, treatment with allopurinol was initiated, 400 mg. daily in four divided doses. By May 1, his nitroglycerine intake had been reduced to four tablets for that week. The patient claimed great improvement, and, when seen on May 15, he had gained six pounds in weight as a result of improved appetite following the complete disappearance of the substernal burning sensation.

CASE 4

A woman of 62, suffering with hypothyroidism, had experienced attacks of angina pectoris since before she was first seen by this investigator in April, 1958. She had been treated with every conceivable drug and drug combination for the relief of her thyroid deficiency, hypercholesterolemia, and cardiac weakness. Most recently, she has been taking digoxin 0.25 mg. and desiccated thyroid 0.065 Gm. Long-acting nitrates had brought very little relief from her anginal attacks. This patient, of normal weight, had the following blood values before commencing allopurinol therapy: serum cholesterol 370 mg. per cent, uric acid 5.6 mg. per cent. Her daily nitroglycerine requirements averaged six tablets daily. On May 29, 1967, she was placed on 600 mg. allopurinol daily. When seen a week later, on June 5, the patient claimed that she felt definitely better and needed only an average of three nitroglycerine tablets daily. On the third day she felt no chest pain whatever and, consequently, did so much work, of the type she was previously unable to perform, that she required five nitroglycerine tablets the following day.

Five additional patients were studied, with similar results, since this paper was prepared.

Discussion

Although the relief of anginal

pain by allopurinol does not prove the plasmalogen theory per se, it was the pursuit of this mechanism which led to the use of the drug. The inferential assumption that allopurinol, by inhibiting xanthine oxidase, increases the blood plasmalogen level is now under investigation. Base values for plasmalogen in the blood will be determined in a larger population group, with all the possible variations owing to drugs, food intake, and age. Allopurinol was designed to inhibit uric acid metabolism. It should be understood that this drug was chosen for use in this investigation only because it was an available nontoxic xanthine oxidase inhibitor. It must surely be realized that there may well be other chemicals with capabilities more specific than that of allopurinol for inhibiting the aldehyde oxidizing qualities of xanthine oxidase. There may also be therapeutic approaches to the restoration of plasmalogen other than inhibition of xanthine oxidase once the plasmalogen theory of angina pectoris and myocardial infarction has found more proof. Angina pectoris and forms of myocardial infarction might be manifestations of plasmalogen diseases, which may also be encountered in other histologic locations of the human body.

The reported difference in plasmalogen distribution between male and female animals and its relationship to gonadal hormones may furnish an explanation of the statistically proven fact that women of childbearing age have such a lower incidence of manifest myocardial infarction than men in the same age

group. Plasmalogens and cholesterol are known components of the cell membrane.[10]

The complex mechanism of pain production in angina pectoris has been ascribed to vascular spasm of the coronary arteries and to production of lactic acid due to poor oxygenation of the myocardial cell. However, neither of these theories explains the pain-relieving action of nitroglycerine in angina pectoris. The theory of plasmalogen depletion in the heart muscle as a possible cause of myocardial pain requires the unopposed action of phospholipase A on plasmalogen according to the equation:

Activated by
Calcium Catecholamines
$\downarrow$
Phospholipase A
$\downarrow$
Plasmalogen
$(+H_2O)$ $\downarrow\uparrow$ $(-H_2O)$
Plasmal + Lysolecithin

Since phospholipase A is an algesic compound, its action without sufficient substrate may be the cause of some of the angina pectoris pain. Restoration of the balance of plasmalogen would then furnish enough substrate for phospholipase A to act on and thus prevent its algesic effect. It is not known if phospholipase A is present in the heart muscle in the form of a proenzyme. It is also not known if nitroglycerine inactivates or neutralizes the activity of phospholipase A. However, it is known that this enzyme may be activated by catechol amines and by calcium ions.

Proceeding with the concept of the outlined theory, the destruction

10. Cuthbert, A. W., *Pharmacol. Rev.*, 19:59-106,1967.

of plasmalogen by xanthine oxidase, occurring normally in the liver, is prevented by the introduction of a xanthine oxidase inhibitor. Allopurinol, a xanthine oxidase inhibitor, was given to patients with known heart disease, and in some patients also hypercholesterolemia, who were sufferers from angina pectoris. There was a definite dosage and response relationship before the angina attacks subsided in frequency and severity. In the language of the proposed theory enough plasmalogen had to be restored to the heart muscle before the action of phospholipase A could be opposed and neutralized. Instead of a diminution of phospholipids in the blood stream which is the aim of most therapeutic endeavors at the present time, an increase of selective phospholipids was here attempted to relieve anginal pain. This was brought about by action on the liver. This organ, when damaged by alcoholic liver cirrhosis, is known to reduce the instance of myocardial infarction by about 80 per cent.[11] Some drugs currently in use for cardiovascular illness act primarily on the liver for their effectiveness, as, for example, the anticoagulants, which alter the prothrombin formed in the liver. Thus, there may well be a relationship of heart to liver in the cause and possible prevention of heart disease. To speculate on the latter, one could visualize a xanthine oxidase activator contained in certain foods as responsible for an excessive destruction of plasmalogen and the cause of eventual myocardial disease.

The four patients studied had no hypertension or obesity, nor have they exhibited hyperuricemia or other manifestations of gout. There are reports that allopurinol-induced reduction of elevated uric acid in the blood of patients with hypercholesteremia and elevated serum triglycerides also caused a reduction of the triglycerides.[12] However, there has been no description of a connection between the action of allopurinol in patients with normal uric acid metabolism and action on the heart, nor have any significant findings of interrelationship of high serum uric acid and angina pectoris been reported.

Summary

A new theory has been postulated as to the cause of some myocardial infarction and angina pectoris. The theory involves an interplay of plasmalogen plus its hydrolysis by phospholipase A to plasmal and lysolecithin. A new therapeutic approach for the treatment of angina pectoris by using xanthine oxidase to inhibit the normal metabolism of plasmalogen in the liver is described. Allopurinol, a xanthine oxidase inhibitor, was successfully used in four cases of angina pectoris to reduce the frequency, duration, and severity of the attacks. A double-blind test was utilized to verify the results obtained. ■

11. Hirst, A. E., et al., *Amer. J. Med. Sci.*, 249:143-149,1965.

12. Berkowitz, D., *J.A.M.A.*, 190:856-858,1964.

Reprinted from Proc. Soc. Exp. Biol. and Med.   Volume 144, Number 2   Nov. 1973
Copyright © 1973 by the Society for Experimental Biology and Medicine   *Printed in U.S.A.*

PROCEEDINGS OF THE SOCIETY FOR EXPERIMENTAL BIOLOGY AND MEDICINE 144,   523–526 (1973)

The Presence of Ectopic Xanthine Oxidase in Atherosclerotic Plaques and Myocardial Tissues[1] (37627)

Donald J. Ross, Michael Ptaszynski,[2] and Kurt A. Oster

Department of Biology, Fairfield University, Fairfield, Connecticut 06430; and Section of Cardiology, Department of Medicine, Park City Hospital, Bridgeport, Connecticut 06604

Plasmalogens, a naturally occurring group of aldehydogenic phospholipids, are found abundantly in human heart and brain tissues. Their phospholipid character makes them an important constituent of many biological membrane systems. Ferrans, Hack, and Borowitz (1) demonstrated plasmalogens in the sarcoplasm, sarcosomes, and intercalate discs of normal human cardiac muscle. Oster and Hope-Ross (2) examined histochemically cardiac muscle from a case of fatal myocardial infarction and found that plasmalogen had disappeared from the infarcted area less than 2 hr after the onset of pain. In this case, there was no necrosis or other significant tissue changes in the affected heart muscle. Similarly, Oster (3) demonstrated the absence of plasmalogen in the aorta of a 22-year-old drowning victim suffering from extensive atherosclerotic changes. Other investigators (4, 5) also demonstrated that plasmalogen depletion in the aortic wall corresponded to an increase in atherosclerosis and that aortic plasmalogen concentrations decreased with age.

It is of significance that certain metabolically active organs—*e.g.*, the liver and mucous membranes of the small intestine—are normally devoid of plasmalogens. Oster and Mulinos (6) ascribed this absence to the activity of the enzyme, xanthine oxidase (xanthine: oxygen oxidoreductase, EC1.2.3.2) which abounds in those tissues where plasmalogen is normally absent. These authors demonstrated that when plasmalogen was split into a fatty aldehyde and lysoplasmalogen by the action of dilute HCl, the resulting aldehydes could be oxidized by purified bovine milk xanthine oxidase preparations. This finding provides a reasonable biochemical explanation for enzyme-mediated plasmalogen depletion. Prior studies by Morgan (7) and Ramboer (8) report the absence of xanthine oxidase in normal human cardiac tissues. The present preliminary investigation endeavors to explain the plasmalogen depletion phenomenon by examining diseased human aortic and myocardial tissues for ectopic xanthine oxidase. No report of the enzyme's presence or absence in diseased tissue has been found in the literature.

Methods. Tissue Sample Selection and Preparation. Unfixed aortic and myocardial tissues of a 54-year-old male and a 74-year-old male were examined (Cases 1 and 2). Their deaths were due to the complications of an abdominal aortic aneurysm and to a myocardial infarction, respectively. In 3 additional cases, the examination for ectopic xanthine oxidase was confined only to the aorta. Case 3 was a 61-year-old male who died from the complications of a bleeding peptic ulcer. He had extensive atherosclerotic calcification of the aortic arch demonstrated by x-ray during life. Case 4 was a 75-year-old male who died from pneumonitis. Calcifications of aorta were examined. Case 5 was a 37-year-old male who died suddenly as a result of a trauma. There was no appreciable amount of atherosclerosis or arteriosclerosis in the aorta.

The entire aortic wall was dissected into little tissue squares (1.0 cm²) visibly containing yellowish atherosclerotic plaques and similar squares of apparently normal, less involved pinkish aortic tissue. The decision for

[1] Supported in part by a research grant from the Greater Bridgeport Chapter of the American Heart Association.

[2] Present address: Hahnemann Medical College, Philadelphia, Pennsylvania.

the myocardial sampling was more difficult because of the lack of a clearly visible demarcation between normal and pathological tissue. Sections near the anterior coronary artery branch were compared with apparently more normal-looking tissue closer to the apex of the heart. Grossly, the latter area showed no evidence of scarring. An average of 8 enzyme assays were performed on homogenates of 2–4 tissue samples from each person.

Estimation of Xanthine Oxidase Activity. Xanthine oxidase activity was measured by the method of Haining and Legan (9). Aortic and myocardial tissue samples were homogenized in 10 vol of cold 0.05 M phosphate buffer (pH 7.4) with EDTA. The homogenate was then centrifuged for 30 min at 4° and 48,000g. The supernatant liquid containing the enzyme was subsequently passed through a Sephadex column (K 9/30) containing G-100 gel which had been pre-irrigated for 1 hr with 0.1 M phosphate buffer (pH 7.4) without EDTA (8). When present, the enzyme would appear in the eluate.

For assay, the reaction mixture consisted of 2.7 ml of 2-amino-4-hydroxypteridine (AHP) in 0.2 M phosphate buffer (pH 7.4) as the substrate and 0.3 ml of the enzyme solution. Appropriate fluorometric blanks were prepared by incubating the buffer substrate and the enzyme solutions in separate test tubes and then combining them after the incubation period and just prior to reading. These blanks and the reaction mixtures were incubated for 1 hr at 37°. Following incubation, 3 ml of impurity-free 40% trichloracetic acid were added to 1 ml portions of both blanks and reaction mixtures. The resulting turbid mixtures were then centrifuged for 10 min at 10,000g to remove precipitated protein. The supernatant fluorescence was measured in a Beckmann Ratio Fluorometer using a number 5 uranium bar, a Schott UG-11 primary filter, and a second Wratten 2A filter. A quinine sulfate solution (1.6 M in 0.1 N sulphuric acid) served as the 100% fluorescence standard.

The unit of enzyme activity was established by the Haining and Legan method, so that each fluorometer scale division measured is equivalent to 1.26×10^{-4} μmoles of AHP

oxidized to the fluorescent product, isoxanthopterin (9). The unit of enzyme activity is expressed as the number of moles of AHP oxidized per g of tissue per hr.

Results. The results (Table I) indicate the presence of xanthine oxidase in many of the samples investigated. As shown, the lowest values for enzyme activity (< 4.69) were observed in aortic tissue samples which appeared grossly normal. Significantly ($p < 0.01$) higher activities were found in samples from both atherosclerotic aortas as well as the pericoronary and apical myocardial tissues of both heart specimens. The variations among the high readings can be ascribed to the differences in severity of the sample pathology, since it is known that tissue reactivity in atherosclerosis and myocardial damage is uneven.

In Cases 3–5, where just the aorta was examined, only one (Case 3) showed ectopic xanthine oxidase in an atherosclerotic lesion. Case 4 with a history of liver disease had no detectable ectopic xanthine oxidase in the lesions examined. The atherosclerotic process in this case showed the severest degree of calcification. Case 5, whose aorta was essentially normal, exhibited no detectable ectopic xanthine oxidase.

Discussion. For the first time, to our knowledge, the presence of xanthine oxidase in the atherosclerotic plaque and the pathological myocardium has been demonstrated. Grossly normal aortic tissues exhibit very little or no detectable enzyme activity, and the same has been reported for normal heart muscle (7, 8). It is possible that this ectopic xanthine oxidase may encounter a suitable substrate in the aldehyde moiety of the phospholipid plasmalogen which is a normal constituent of the cell membranes of such tissues. The subsequent alteration of the structural integrity of these membranes by such enzymatic activity may produce an initial lesion which could then serve to increase cell permeability, microthrombus deposition, or both.

One source of the enzyme may be the liver cell, since patients with acute liver disease show increased serum levels of xanthine oxidase (8). In patients with chronic liver disease, the serum level of xanthine oxidase

XANTHINE OXIDASE IN ATHEROSCLEROSIS

TABLE I. Xanthine Oxidase Activity in Normal and Pathological Human Aortic and Myocardial Tissue Homogenates.

Male patient no.	Age	Tissue sampling	Samples (n)	Mean g tissue/ml homogenate	Mean moles AHP[a] oxidized/hr	Xanthine oxidase activity[a]
1	54	Normal-appearing aorta (control)	3	0.320	$1.89 \times 10^{-4} \pm 0.04$	4.69 ± 0.10
1		Atherosclerotic aorta	4	0.493	$5.56 \times 10^{-4} \pm 0.08$	89.5 ± 0.36
2	74	Normal-appearing aorta (control)	2	0.289	$<5.6 \times 10^{-4}$[b]	
2		Atherosclerotic plaque (aorta)	3	0.239	$1.01 \times 10^{-4} \pm 0.07$	33.5 ± 2.3
1		Normal-appearing myocardium (control)	2	0.220	♦	
2		Normal-appearing myocardium (control)	2	0.244		
1		Pericoronary myocardium of right lateral branch of coronary artery	2	0.301	$2.48 \times 10^{-4} \pm 0.04$	65.3 ± 10.8
2		Area from apex of heart with no visible epicardial scarring	3	0.332	$1.10 \times 10^{-4} \pm 0.06$	26.3 ± 1.4
3	61	Atherosclerotic aorta	3	0.249	$7.02 \times 10^{-4} \pm 0.14$	28.19 ± 2.7
4	75	Atherosclerotic aorta	3	0.314	♦	
5	37	Normal aorta (control)	3	0.219		

[a] Moles of 2-amino-4-hydroxypteridine (AHP) oxidized/g tissue/hr. An average of 8 enzyme assays were performed on each tissue sample. Results are expressed as averages ± SD.

[b] Minimal detectable activity level for method employed.

is occasionally moderately elevated. Moreover, in uncomplicated, obstructive jaundice, the serum xanthine oxidase is, at times, slightly elevated (8). In addition to these findings, Ramboer (8) was able to demonstrate slight xanthine oxidase activity in the sera of 10 out of 25 normal human subjects, although Shamma'a et al. (10) detected no xanthine oxidase activity in the sera of 18 healthy subjects. Another potential source of the enzyme, viz. bovine milk ingestion, is presently under investigation in this laboratory, since it has been shown that milk antibodies are significantly elevated in the blood of male patients with ischaemic heart disease (11).

The postulated enzyme-induced alteration of the phospholipid composition of the cell membrane may point to ectopic xanthine oxidase as one of the factors inducing serious inflammation or perfusion of the arterial endothelium or the myocardium as described by Haust (12). Roussos (13) has shown that bovine xanthine oxidase activity is stimulated by androsterone and testosterone and inhibited by the estrogens (β-estradiol, 17α-estradiol, estrone, and estriol) and progesterone. This could account for the predominance of atherosclerotic heart disease in men.

Summary. Xanthine oxidase activity of five grossly normal aortic tissues of five male patients was compared with that of atheromas from the same aortas. In addition, pathological myocardial tissues of two of the patients were examined. Significantly elevated enzyme activities were found in most abnormal tissue samples. Little or no activity was detected in the normal-appearing samples. These results suggest that xanthine oxidase may be deposited gradually with time, possibly initiating a pathological reaction which culminates in plaque formation or myocardial cellular damage.

1. Ferrans, V. J., Hack, M. H., and Borowitz, E. H. J., Histochem. Cytochem. 10, 462 (1962).

2. Oster, K. A., and Hope-Ross, P., Amer. J. Cardiol. 17, 83 (1966).

3. Oster, K. A., Amer. J. Clin. Res. 2, 30 (1971).

4. Buddecke, E., and Andresen, G., Hoppe Seiler's Z. Physiol. Chem. 314, 38 (1959).

5. Miller, B., Anderson, C. E., and Piantadosi, C. J., Gerontology 19, 430 (1964).

6. Oster, K. A., and Mulinos, M. G., J. Pharmacol. Exp. Ther. 80, 132 (1944).

7. Morgan, E. J., Biochem. J. 161, 1280 (1926).

8. Ramboer, C. R. H., J. Lab. Clin. Med. 74, 828 (1969).

9. Haining, J. L., and Legan, J. S., Anal. Biochem. 21, 337 (1967).

10. Shamma'a, M. H., Gastroenterology 48, 226 (1965).

11. Davies, D. F., J. Atheroscler. Res. 9, 103 (1969).

12. Haust, M. D., and More, R. H., in "The Pathogenesis of Atherosclerosis" (R. W. Wissler and J. C. Greer, eds.), p. 11. Williams and Wilkins Co., Baltimore (1972).

13. Roussos, G. G., Biochim. Biophys. Acta 73, 338 (1963).

Received April 24, 1973. P.S.E.B.M., 1973, Vol. 144.

CLINICAL ⧗ PERSPECTIVES

Is an Enzyme in Homogenized Milk the Culprit in Dietary-Induced Atherosclerosis?

Kurt A. Oster, M.D.

Certain findings developed in the last thirty years may explain the dietary origin of atherosclerosis. The acceptance of Plasmalogen Disease as partially caused by dietary xanthine oxidase from cows' milk would make it possible to prevent this cause of atherosclerosis with a simple dietary modification. For atherosclerotic lesions still amenable to treatment, a method of treatment is proposed making use of folic acid's known biochemical inhibition of xanthine oxidase.

This new concept runs counter to prevailing dietary dogma, which advises avoiding saturated fats and cholesterol to reduce atherosclerotic lesions and myocardial infarction, a belief that culminated in the Inter-Society Report on the Prevention of Atherosclerotic Disease (1970).

Problem

The Masai, who ingest an inordinate amount of milk and saturated fatty acids, are a stumbling

---

Dr. Oster is a Fellow of the American College of Physicians, the American College of Cardiology, and the American College for Clinical Pharmacology.

block to the theory that maintains milk and fatty acids are the major cause of hypercholesterolemia and atherosclerosis. Despite their diet, the rarity of atherosclerosis among these East African cattle herders invalidates animal experiments involving unnatural diets causing storage diseases of unassimilable foreign lipids. Yet those who embrace the hypercholesterolemia theory seek and find every excuse to sidestep this nutritional reality in humans.

The latest attempt to sustain the hypercholesterolemia theory (Ho, *et al*, 1971) ascribes a specific genetic trait to these pastoral people. In this experiment, 23 young Masai were observed, 11 serving as controls with a base line serum cholesterol of 126 mg percent, and 12 serving as an experimental group with 124 mg percent serum cholesterol. But these cholesterol levels were unstable. After eight weeks, values rose to 175 mg percent and 170 mg percent respectively, a 39 percent and a 43 percent increase. This counterindicates a genetic trait of cholesterol feedback and demonstrates the futility of drawing conclusions from small numbers and unproven assumptions.

Others have stated that paucity of atherosclerosis in the Masai stems from physical exercise and lack of emotional stress (Mann, 1964). But the lumber-producing natives of East Finland expend more energy in woodchopping than do the Masai in herding. Despite intense physical activity, the Finns suffer the world's highest death rate from myocardial infarction.

Applying the concept of Plasmalogen Disease caused by biologically available xanthine oxidase in cows' milk, no excuses need be made regarding the rarity of atheroscloisis in the Masai. Nor must we exclude them from the human community in favor of findings in baboons, chickens, rabbits, or rats. Nutritional facts observed in Nature's experiment with this tribe explain, without exception or subterfuge, the scarcity of atherosclerosis.

Mechanism

The new concept of Plasmalogen Disease deals with an essential component of the cell membrane, a phospholipid, named "Plasmalogen" by its discoverers (Feulgen and Voit) in 1924.

Plasmalogen is widely distributed in the human body, with highest concentrations in skeletal muscle, cardiac muscle, the intima of the arterial wall, and the myelin sheath of nerve tissue. Normal liver tissue of most animals and humans is devoid of plasmalogen, but contains xanthine oxidase, an aldehyde-oxidizing enzyme. Oster and Mulinos (1945) proved that the absence of one is due to the presence of the other.

Several authors have described the absence of plasmalogen from atherosclerotic plaque: Buddecke and Andresen in 1959; Miller, Anderson, and Piantadosi in 1964; and Oster in 1971. Absence of plasmalogen from heart muscle tissue, in a case of fatal myocardial infarction before cell death, was reported by Oster and Hope-Ross in 1966. Lack of plasmalogen was demonstrated in the demyelinated lesion of multiple sclerosis (Gerstl, *et al*, 1962).

Plasmalogen Disease is a newly created term applied to pathological plasmalogen deficiencies with specific expressions or manifestations, depending on anatomical sites.

Without doubt, something in the human diet causes early atherosclerosis. The search for the 'something' seemed to have ended in the United

States in December, 1970, when the Inter-Society Report on the Prevention of Atherosclerotic Diseases recommended changing the amounts of saturated fats and cholesterol in the American diet. Proponents feel that lowering serum cholesterol in this manner greatly reduces myocardial infarction. Commission members claim people in economically developed countries consume more saturated fats and cholesterol than do people in high carbohyrate-consuming, less economically advanced nations.

This statement has a hollow ring. Kahn (1970) proved that the intake of saturated fats in the United States was the same with early 1900's pork-eating generations as it is with the present beef-consuming population. And though milk consumption by North American adults has decreased, atherosclerotic disease manifestations have increased. Again the Masai fail to fit this configuration, although they consume enormous amounts of saturated fats.

Despite the differential, a common element in the diet to both the Masai and North Americans is cows' milk. In fact, cows' milk is the only important food containing xanthine oxidase that is consumed by people of many nations. Oddly enough, human milk lacks this enzyme.

In a table of death rates from coronary heart disease and dairy product consumption in thirteen economically developed nations, the United States ranks ninth in milk consumption, eleventh in butter intake, and seventh in cheese consumption. Yet the United States has the second highest myocardial infarction death rate in men aged 45–54 years. The Masai, with 66 percent of their calories provided by fat, have very little atherosclerosis. Why the paradox?

The paradox lies in the fact that a physical characteristic of cows' milk has changed in this century in the United States. With universal homogenization, particle size of fats and proteins in milk emulsion is less than one micron. This minute particle size permits xanthine oxidase to pass through the intestinal barrier. By way of the lymph stream, it may then enter the arterial system, depositing itself in arterial walls and the heart muscle. This provides a rational biochemical explanation of plasmalogen depletion caused by xanthine oxidase. Plasmalogen depletion results in atherosclerosis and myocardial damage, depending on the local tissue repair mechanism. It follows that *the dietary origin of the atherosclerotic lesion is proportional to the biological availability of xanthine oxidase in youth.*

Prevention

Atherosclerosis caused by xanthine oxidase in homogenized milk is a disease of male and female youth. Therefore, it should be prevented in youth, not in the 30 to 40 age group, as is so often recommended. Prevention lies in the creation of a milk containing no biologically available xanthine oxidase. This occurs when milk is boiled, or when the particle size permits xanthine oxidase to be digested, not absorbed.

It appears that the healthiest way to consume milk is either by preboiling, as practiced by Europeans with a low heart attack rate, or by consuming it in curdled form, as do the economically backward Masai. Without resorting to genetic traits, we now have a plausible explanation for the paucity of atherosclerosis among East African cattle herders.

Treatment

Treatment of dietary-induced atherosclerosis can be accomplished only when active ectopic xanthine oxidase is still present in tissues. One cannot expect an established calcified lesion to respond to any treatment other than surgical replacement. It is preferable, in searching for a xanthine oxidase inhibitor, to find one harmless in large doses to humans. A past study utilized allopurinol, a synthetic oxidase inhibitor. Because of its potential toxicity in prolonged use, it was not recommendable (Oster, 1968). It has been stated that pteridines are xanthine oxidase inhibitors (Kalckar, Kjeldfaard, and Klenow, 1950). Curiously enough, they have never been used for this purpose in humans.

Since xanthine oxidase converts xanthine and hypoxanthine to uric acid in human purine metabolism, patients with hyperuricemia were chosen as test objects in an in vivo investigation of folic (pteroyl glutamic) acid inhibition. The desired effect would be a significant lowering of the serum uric acid level in hyperuricemic patients. In vitro experiments established that the dosage level needed by a person of average weight should be between 40 and 80 mg of folic acid.

All sixteen cases of hyperuricemia responded well. High uric acid levels were lowered to normal ranges with folic acid therapy, a level maintainable for twelve months. Cessation of treatment resulted in hyperuricemia.

Once the xanthine oxidase-inhibiting quality of folic acid was established in vivo, the next step was to examine the effect of large pharmacological doses of folic acid on visible atherosclerotic lesions. Elderly diabetics were chosen for this purpose. Patients with ulceration and ischemic discoloration of the toes were given 80 mg folic acid daily in divided doses. After three weeks of therapy, lesions which had been resistant to treatment with every known modality improved noticeably.

No experience with multiple sclerosis has been gathered. Trial treatments with folic acid are being given to cases of generalized atherosclerosis and coronary atherosclerosis. However, in contrast to many studies of 50 to 60 year old institutionalized men, no parameters or predictive criteria exist to say with certainty that a person is free of atherosclerosis, with or without treatment. Serum cholesterol levels and their potential reduction are not acceptable as evidence of successful therapeutic intervention. However, treatment with folic acid is being continued. Hopefully, a report on results with forty persons now under observation will be shortly forthcoming.

Discussion

Atherosclerosis investigation suffers because no suitable model exists for demonstrating successful prevention or treatment of atherosclerotic lesions. Animal experiments are unsuitable because toxic effects caused by drugs or dietary manipulation are often reversible when toxic substances are withdrawn. Disappearance of so-called atherosclerotic lesions, or withdrawal of lesion-producing diets in a test animal, do not establish a mechanism of cause and prevention. The arbiter of success or failure, both for prevention and therapy, should be the human atherosclerotic lesion.

A single plasmalogen disease manifestation may serve as a desired model, provided one assumes a uniform cause and a multiform expression of the disease. Similar conditions are encountered in most diseases where a single organism, invading normal tissues, evokes many different, apparently unrelated disease expressions. Infection with Treponema pallidum may cause aortitis, gummata, bone changes, or a tabes doralis-like neurological disease, according to the tissue invaded. Such may be the case with xanthine oxidase-caused plasmalogen depletion. A multitude of apparently unrelated diseases may actually be only one many-faceted disease. Hopefully, these manifestations will be amenable to one treatment.

Pharmacological doses of folic acid may be the uniform therapy for plasmalogen diseases. In this respect, amazing therapeutic responses of hyperuricemia and peripheral atherosclerotic lesions are encouraging. Hopefully, other investigators will try this newly devised therapy with similar results.

Summary

Prevention of dietary atherosclerosis may lie in avoiding biologically available xanthine oxidase in cows' milk. This can be accomplished either by destroying the enzyme through heat, or by creating particles in the food which are large enough to be digested, not absorbed.

Treatment of existing lesions consists of pharmacological doses of folic acid, a well-known xanthine oxidase inhibitor. Because the Masai consume milk in a form with large-sized particles, without biologically available xanthine oxidase, they are protected from dietary-induced atherosclerosis. If encroaching 'civilization' induces the Masai to relinquish their way of life and consume milk with the additive of biologically available xanthine oxidase, this situation may be reversed.

Acknowledgements

My thanks to Dr. D. J. Ross of Fairfield University, Fairfield, Conn., in whose laboratory were performed the in vitro studies of folic acid inhibition of xanthine oxidase.

By Kurt A. Oster, Jeffrey B. Oster, and Donald J. Ross

Immune response to bovine xanthine oxidase in atherosclerotic patients

K NOWLEDGE OF the etiology of the atherosclerotic process is virtually nonexistent, and because of this lack of knowledge the prevention and treatment of atherosclerosis is in a deplorable state. The problem is importunate; hence, potentially dangerous pseudosolutions based on expediency and temporizing are offered. A tenuous association of elevated serum cholesterol found in certain homogeneous population groups is made the fulcrum of a therapeutic approach by diet and drugs for the reduction of risk of the sequelae of atherosclerotic involvement. Grandiose schemes for serum cholesterol reduction in the prevention and treatment of atherosclerotic coronary heart disease have wide semiofficial sanction by government institutions and voluntary health organizations. Curiously enough, the same approach of serum cholesterol reduction is seldom advocated in the treatment of peripheral artery atherosclerosis, found mainly in the atherosclerotic brain syndrome and the ischemic lesions of the lower extremities affecting so many diabetic patients.[1]

A new theory of the genesis of the atherosclerotic process has been postulated.[2] In essence it claims that the dietary origin of this disease is initiated by the absorption through the intestinal wall of xanthine oxidase contained in bovine milk and that the enzyme is then carried by the lymph stream to the arterial vascular system and hence deposited by an insudative process into the vessel walls and the myocardium. In these ectopic sites xanthine oxidase alters the integrity of the cell membrane by oxidizing a phospholipid, plasmalogen. The resulting pathological processes have been named Plasmalogen Diseases, with specific pathological manifestations in different anatomical sites.

This theory has been attacked as nonviable because of a traditional belief that a large molecule such as xanthine oxidase (molecular weight 290,000) cannot be absorbed intact; and, consequently, presence of xanthine oxidase in ectopic locations[3] could not derive from bovine milk but could originate only from such endogenous sources as the intestine or the liver.

The present study is concerned with this problem of intestinal absorption of large protein molecules from dietary sources. Preliminary demonstration of such absorption has been forthcoming in many reports. One finds a summary of these findings in a publication by Davies.[4] Davies has also shown by specific hemagglutination of sensitized sheep blood cells that milk proteins were absorbed into the human bloodstream. In addition, he found that patients with ischemic heart disease had a higher, statistically significant, antibody level to milk proteins than patients without the symptoms of ischemic heart disease.

We attempted to duplicate Davies's findings in patients with manifest atherosclerotic diseases, such as coronary heart disease, atherothrombotic brain syndrome, and peripheral atherosclerosis (claudication and threatening gangrene). We expanded his study to include not only milk proteins but also specific antibodies to xanthine oxidase from bovine sources. It was hoped that results of this study would demonstrate conclusively that this enzyme is absorbed, as postulated, and that eventual antibodies to it could be traced through the various age groups, despite the fact that milk intake in

Dr. K. Oster is Chief of Cardiology, Park City Hospital, and Adjunct Research Professor of Biology, Fairfield University; Mr. J. Oster is presently Senior Premedical Student, Johns Hopkins University, and was formerly the recipient of a summer research grant from the Greater Bridgeport Heart Association; Dr. Ross is Professor of Biology, Fairfield University.

The authors thank Barbara B. O'Neill R.N. and C. Brian Cheney F.I.M.L.T. for their valuable assistance.

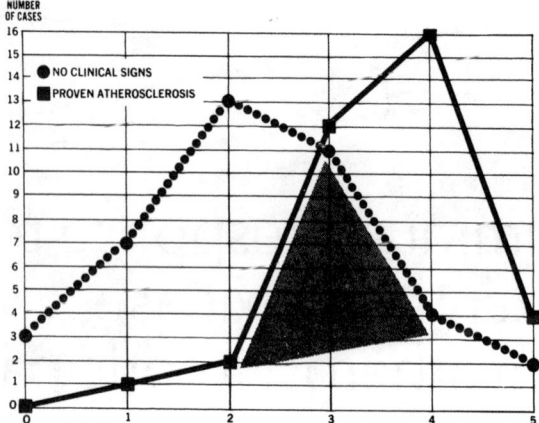

Figure 1 *Immunoassay of serum xanthine oxidase.*

adults is negligible compared with its greater consumption in youth.

Methods

Two separate antibody titrations were performed on each blood sample: a milk antibody test followed the method of Rees,[5] and xanthine oxidase antibodies were determined by an adaptation of the Boyden tanned erythrocyte technique.[6]

All solutions were prepared as described in Refs. 5 and 6, with one exception: the human sera were mixed with buffered saline in geometric 1:1 serial dilution instead of the neutral rabbit serum used by Rees. For the xanthine oxidase antibody test a 0.5% protein solution with sigma grade 2 xanthine oxidase* in 2.3 M ammonium sulfate solution was prepared by dilution (1:20) with 66.7% buffered saline and 33.3% of 0.66 M phosphate buffer (pH 7.4). Care was taken to ensure proper osmolarity for the sheep red blood cells.

Agglutination was measured on a scale of 0 to 5 by halves as an expression of each geometric dilution. A reading of 0 showed no agglutination, and a value of 5+ represented the highest antibody concentration measured.

Every investigated blood serum showed sequential agglutination. There was no pro-zone, and no serial dilution of the sera failed to show agglutination.

Controls

Control experiments were performed to rule out nonspecific agglutinations. A buffered saline solu-

tion that was added to the sensitized red sheep cells did not result in any agglutination. It was considered a negative control. A positive control was employed and consisted of unwashed, unsensitized sheep red blood cells diluted (1:60) with buffered saline to which was added an equal volume of undiluted, complement-inactivated serum.

Several sera were tested with both active xanthine oxidase antigen and heat-inactivated xanthine oxidase antigen. The antibody-antigen reaction was the same in both test groups. This finding supports the claim by Ultmann, Feigelson, and Harris[7] that the antigenic property of heat-inactivated xanthine oxidase is no less than that of active xanthine oxidase. Nevertheless, only further tests will prove if this important finding is reproducible in all specimens. Further, there must be a delineation of the limitations of the inactivation of xanthine oxidase before a possible screening of patients with inactivated xanthine oxidase can be initiated.

Patient material

Patients were selected at random by a registered nurse from an office practice of internal medicine. Under double-blind conditions the bloods were consecutively numbered, and none of the investigators was aware of the identity of any blood sample. When all tests were completed, the patients were divided into two groups by the senior author. (K. Oster) according to one criterion: presence or absence of clinical manifestations of atherosclerotic disease. These manifestations embraced all varieties of atherosclerosis, such as angina pectoris, myocardial infarction, serious cardiac arrhythmias, claudication, peripheral vascular disease with threatening gangrene, and atherosclerotic brain syndrome. Hypertensive and rheumatic valvular heart disease patients were considered as nonatherosclerotic for the purpose of the study.

---

*Sigma grade IV xanthine oxidase solution contains 112 mg protein/ml.

IMMUNE RESPONSE

Results

The test group of 75 patient sera revealed varying titers of specific antibodies to bovine xanthine oxidase. Neither age nor sex exerted any apparent influence on the response. The study comprised 47 males and 28 females, whose ages ranged from 21 to 90 years. Surprisingly both the 21- and the 90-year old had high xanthine oxidase agglutination responses.

Figure 1 shows the frequency distribution of the various agglutination values found in the atherosclerotic and nonatherosclerotic patient groups. The abscissa indicates the various degrees of agglutination, 1+ through 5+. The ordinate lists the number of cases involved. The dotted line represents those patients with no detectable signs of atherosclerosis and the solid line the manifest atherosclerotics. Fractional values were rounded out to the next higher full value.

Two peaks are visible in the frequency distribution of the nonatherosclerotic and atherosclerotic groups. The nonatherosclerotics have mostly a 2+ agglutination reaction (13 cases) and a weak 3+ reaction (11 cases). The atherosclerotics show a peak agglutination of 4+ (16 cases) and 3+ (12 cases). The two groups overlap in a gray area between 2+ and 4+ agglutination. One may speculate that the group with no clinical manifestations of atherosclerosis may well have atherosclerotic lesions somewhere in their bodies which have not yet attained detectable status. On the other hand, those patients with known atherosclerosis who responded with low agglutination values may be the ones with poor general immunity. These were mostly people with thyroid deficiency.

Tables 1 and *2* list the individual test subjects and their agglutination responses (degree of antibody production) to milk proteins and to bovine xanthine oxidase. Scrutiny of a few individual cases reveals some interesting observations. A 47-year-old nonpatient, recruited as an apparently healthy person, had a 5+ xanthine oxidase agglutination response. When questioned about her milk history, she revealed that for many years the presence of a peptic ulcer had necessitated a diet high in cream and milk. Despite subsequent subtotal gastrectomy she had continued for two years her substantial intake of milk and cream.

Two young healthy Italian immigrants appeared for a required premarital blood test. Both had only 1+ agglutination. Their milk history revealed that the 24-year-old bride had been drinking only goat's milk most of her life, and the groom, a country boy, had been given only raw unrefrigerated cow's milk.

It is known that raw untreated and unrefrigerated milk contains very little biologically available xanthine oxidase.[8]

Two natives of India were tested. Both were accustomed to drink boiled buffalo milk in their native land. The 28-year-old husband had a 1+ xanthine oxidase agglutination response, the 22-year old wife a 5+ agglutination. She suffers with chronic gastroenteritis and has been ingesting large quantities of homogenized cow's milk since living in this country.

In all likelihood absorption of foreign proteins through the damaged intestinal mucosa differs from absorption through the intact mucous membrane. One may well wonder how increase in penetrability of foreign proteins is enhanced by such commonly used drugs as acetyl salicylic acid, ethyl alcohol, emulsifiers, and detergents. It is hoped that these potential interactions of drugs and chemicals on our food utilization and absorption will be investigated and determined.

This study has led to one unavoidable conclusion. Bovine xanthine oxidase must have been absorbed through the intestinal wall, because specific antibodies to the enzyme were demonstrated in human sera. The major objection to the theory of the genesis of atherosclerotic lesions by absorbed xanthine oxidase has thereby been effectively countered.

Independent t tests were performed on the data for antibodies to both xanthine oxidase and to milk to determine whether significant differences existed between the groups. A total of 75 cases were tested for 75 degrees of freedom. The antibody-to-milk-protein test had an independent t value of 2.89, and so $p < 0.01$, which is very significant. Coincidently Davies obtained an independent t value of 2.85 in 50 cases with 48 degrees of freedom. The antibodies-to-xanthine-oxidase test had an independent t value of 4.86, and so $p < 0.001$, which is extremely significant.

The statistical significance of finding higher xanthine oxidase antibodies in test subjects with demonstrable atherosclerotic manifestations than in those with no clinical evidence of the disease should be submitted to further extensive testing. If confirmed by our ongoing investigation and by others, it could be developed into an important screening test. One might say that an individual with an antibody reaction of 3+ or higher would have atherosclerotic processes initiated by xanthine oxidase somewhere in his body. The location would have to be determined by more intensive examination. Such a test would be a vast improvement over the so often meaningless (because of its variability) serum cholesterol determination.

It is not known if a high level of antibody to xanthine oxidase is beneficial or harmful to the individual. We have opted for the former position. Ultmann et al.[7] have found that antibodies to xanthine oxidase inhibit the activity of the enzyme up to 70% because of noncompetitive antibody-antigen binding. One might then assume that antibodies to bovine xanthine oxidase are the body's defense mechanism against persistent ectopically depcsited bovine xanthine oxidase. The argument that the ectopically found enzyme originates from the liver or the intestine is invalid according to our study, in which we have found close correlation between the antibody level and increased bovine milk intake. Additionally, the differences between milk antibody and xanthine oxidase antibody responses by the same test individual would not have occurred, had the enzyme originated from autogenous human sources.

One of the most unexpected findings in this study was the observation that patients up to 90 years of age still have measurable antibodies to bovine xanthine oxidase in their sera. This demonstration together with the published finding[3] of active xanthine oxidase in atherosclerotic plaques and myocardial tissue in elderly patients should serve as a major stepping-stone to the experimental proof of the origin of the atherosclerotic lesion, that of bovine xanthine oxidase attacking plasmalogen in the cell membrane, a pathological process which has been termed plasmalogen disease.

References

1. GORDON, T. and KANNEL, W. B., "Predisposition to atherosclerosis in the head, heart, and legs: The Framingham study," *J.A.M.A. 221*, 661–666 (1972).
2. OSTER, K. A., "Plasmalogen diseases. A new concept of the etiology of the atherosclerotic process," *Amer. J. Clin. Res. 2*, 30–35 (1971); OSTER, K. A., "Role of plasmalogen in heart diseases," *Myocardiology*, edited by E. Bajusz and G. Rona, (University Park Press, Baltimore, 1972), vol. 1, pp. 803–813; OSTER, K. A., "Evaluation of serum cholesterol reduction and xanthine oxidase inhibition in the treatment of atherosclerosis," *Myocardial Metabolism*, edited by N. S. Dhalla, (University Park Press, Baltimore, 1973), pp. 73–80.
3. ROSS, D. J., PTASZYNSKI, M., and OSTER, K. A., "The presence of ectopic xanthine oxidase in atherosclerotic plaques and myocardial tissues," *Proc. Soc. Exp. Biol. Med., 144*, 523–526 (1973).
4. DAVIES, D. F., DAVIES, J. R., and RICHARDS, M. A., "Antibodies to reconstituted dried cows milk protein in coronary heart disease," *J. Atherscl. Res. 9*, 103–107 (1969).
5. REES, B. N. G., "An automated method for the coated tanned red cell hemagglutination technique," *Med. Lab. Tech. 30*, 167–177 (1973).
6. BOYDEN, S. J., "The adsorption of proteins on erythrocytes treated with tannic acid and subsequent hemagglutination by antiprotein sera," *J. Exp. Med. 93*, 107–120 (1951).
7. ULTMANN, J. E., FEIGELSON, P., and HARRIS, S., "The effect of specific antibodies on xanthine oxidase from various sources," *J. Immun. 88*, 113–117 (1962).
8. ROBERT, L. and POLONOVSKY, J., "Activation and inactivation of milk xanthine oxidase by physicochemical means," *Disc. Faraday Soc. 20*, 54–65 (1955).

Recent Advances in Studies on
Cardiac Structure and Metabolism Volume 10
The Metabolism of Contraction
Edited by Paul-Emile Roy and George Rona
Copyright 1975   University Park Press   Baltimore

AN ENZYME MECHANISM IN EXPLANATION
OF PAIN IN ANGINA PECTORIS

KURT A. OSTER and DONALD J. ROSS

Department of Biology, Fairfield University,
Fairfield, Connecticut, USA

SUMMARY

The effect of catecholamines, represented by epinephrine and norepinephrine, on the activity of phospholipase A_2 from bee venom was studied. It was shown that the hydrolysis of l-α-lecithin to lysolecithin and a fatty acid was considerably activated by preincubation of the lecithin with the biogenic amine. On the other hand, addition of nitroglycerin or propranolol to the enzyme solution considerably curtailed activation by the catecholamines. The pharmacological effect of the split products of l-α-lecithin, free fatty acids (FFA), and lysolecithin in the nascent state on the myocardial cell membrane might be more plausible than the commonly accepted theory that the FFA derive from lipolysis of remote fat deposits. Certain arrhythmias and ion imbalances might be caused by catecholamine activation of phospholipase A_2. Of great pharmacological interest is the observation that this activation is inhibited by a beta-adrenergic blocking agent without the presence of cyclic adenosine monophosphate as messenger. The reaction may serve as a model for the study of the pharmacological influence of nitroglycerin and propranolol on angina pectoris.

INTRODUCTION

The cause of the pain experienced in angina pectoris is unknown. An attempt had been made to attribute the pain sensation experienced during angina pectoris attacks to the action of myocardial phospholipase A_2 (E.C.3.1.1.4) on cell membrane-associated phospholipids (Oster, 1968). The authors, recalling the known algesic effect of subcutaneously injected bee venom, which consists mainly of phospholipases, have postulated that a similar enzyme, situated in the myocardial cell, might also effect pain when triggered by such stimuli of heart action as emotion, mild exertion, heavy meals, and nonspecific stimuli which might occur during sleep.

In a published schematic approach to the metabolism of plasmalogen (Oster, 1972), the enzyme phospholipase A_2 was shown to be activated by Ca^{++} ions and catecholamines. At that time, literature describing calcium activation of the enzyme had been reviewed by Meldrum (1965). However, the postulated activation of phospholipase A_2 by catecholamines had never been described before the schematics were published. Feeling that such a significant clue to the origin of pain in heart muscle merited a thorough inquiry, we set out to investigate this postulated catecholamine activation of phospholipase A_2, hoping that such a study might also provide additional insight into the pharmacological effects of two categories of antianginal drugs, nitrites (nitroglycerin) and the beta-receptor blockers (propranolol).

The effects on lipid metabolism of injected catecholamines have thus far been tested in the intact animal or the open-chest animal preparation (Opie, 1972). In order to learn more about the basic mechanism, we preferred to use the pure enzyme in bee venom as a cell-free model, thus eliminating such extraneous influences as foreign proteins and fats, morphological structures, and the presence of other amine-inactivating enzymes.

It is understood that this approach may not be entirely applicable to the biochemical metabolism of the mammalian myocardium. Nevertheless, as will be shown in the "Discussion," we know that the cyclic AMP-mediated, lipolytic action of injected catecholamines liberates large amounts of free fatty acids (FFA) in the test animal. Combined with plasma protein, this reaction may well mask the pharmacological effects of the FFA arising from the action of phospholipase A_2, situated in the myocardial cell, on its substrate, the phospholipids. We thought that these cardiogenic FFA in their nascent state might possess more pharmacological significance than those which are transported through the circulatory system after liberation. Many investigators have reported conflicting results from FFA obtained through lipolytic action of the catecholamines (Opie, 1972). Our *in vitro* test method has also enabled us to vary the amounts of catecholamines within their physiological range without fear that other metabolic systems may trap them and make them unavailable.

METHOD

Enzymatic assay of phospholipase A_2 derived from bee venom

Reaction: Lecithin + H_2O $\xrightarrow{\text{Phospho-lipase } A_2}$ Lysolecithin + an unsaturated fatty acid ion.

Unit definition: 1 unit will cleave 1 μmole of l-α-lecithin to lysolecithin and a fatty acid in 1 min at $37°C$ at pH 6.6.

Method of assy: Colorimetric at 570 mμ, pH 6.6, $37°C$, based primarily on the method of Magee and Thompson (1960) as modified by Dawson (1963). This measures the decrease of lecithin and is based on the ability of carboxylic ester groups in intact lipids to react with hydroxylamine in alkaline solution to yield hydroxamic acids. The hydroxamic acids react with ferric chloride to give colored ferric hydroxamic acid complexes.

Reagents
Buffer: 0.5 M Tris, pH 6.6
Substrate: 20 mg/ml lecithin in 0.01 M calcium chloride
Activator: 1.5% sodium deoxycholate
Other: 3:1 v/v ethanol:ethyl ether
2 M hydroxylamine HCl
14% NaOH
3 N HCl
10% anhydrous ferric chloride in 0.1 N HCl
Enzyme: Diluted in 50% glycerol to give 2 units/ml
Reaction mixture: 1) 0.7 ml lecithin emulsion, 20 mg/ml
2) 0.7 ml 0.5 M buffer, pH 6.6
3) 0.7 ml 1.5% sodium deoxycholate (warm to 37°C)
4) 0.1 ml diluted enzyme (approximately 0.2 unit)

Physiological concentrations
Activators of
phospholipase A_2:

Epinephrine, 0.01 μg/100 ml
Norephinephrine, 0.05 μg/100 ml, added to reaction mixture 5 min before enzyme

Inhibitors of
activated phospho-
lipase A_2:

Nitroglycerin, 2.4 $\times$ 10^{-5} mg/ml
Propranolol, 1.0 μg/ml, added with enzyme

RESULTS

Findings in the catecholamine-activated cleavage of phosphatidylcholine by phospholipase A_2 and its partial curtailment by nitroglycerin and propranolol are depicted in Figures 1–3 (a more detailed description of the results will be published elsewhere).

Figure 1 shows the considerable activation of phospholipase A_2 by epinephrine (0.01 μg/100 ml) and the influence of nitroglycerin (2.4$\times$10^{-5} mg/ml) on this effect. In 5 min, 8.44 μmoles of l-α-lecithin were hydrolyzed. This value was reduced to 6.65 μmoles by the action of nitroglycerin.

As is seen in Figure 2, the norepinephrine activation of phospholipase A_2 in 5 min to 9.63 μmoles (an increase over the normal 6.14 μmoles) was significantly

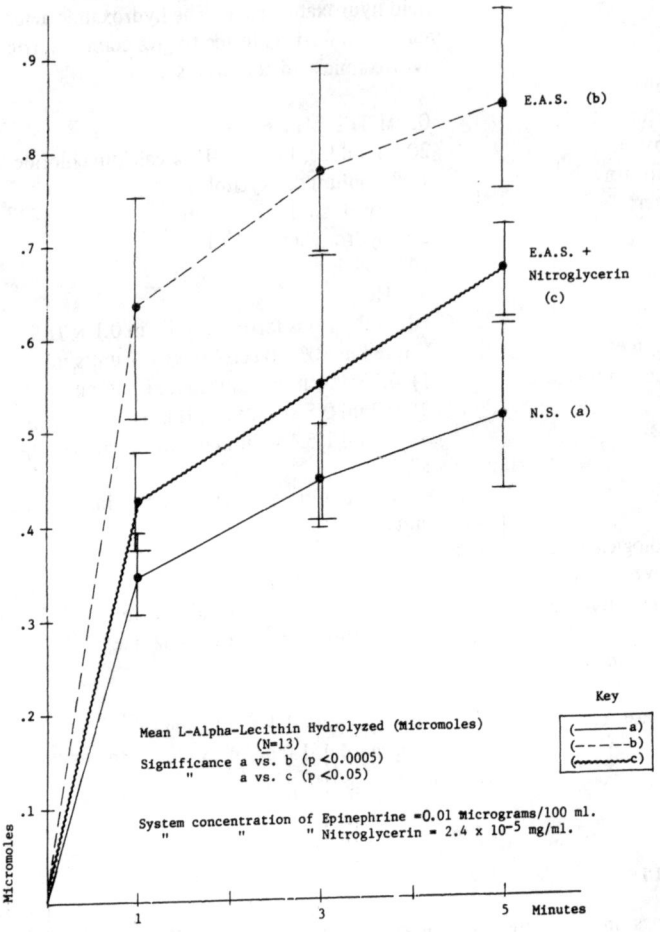

Key

(————)	a)
(— — — —)	b)
(∿∿∿∿∿)	c)

Mean L-Alpha-Lecithin Hydrolyzed (micromoles)
(N=13)
Significance a vs. b (p <0.0005)
"   a vs. c (p <0.05)

System concentration of Epinephrine = 0.01 micrograms/100 ml.
"   "   " Nitroglycerin = 2.4 x 10⁻⁵ mg/ml.

Figure 1. Epinephrine-activated phospholipase A_2 with nitroglycerin deactivation.

reduced by nitroglycerin to 6.20 umoles, which approximates the normal hydrolysis.

Propranolol effects were studied thus far only in the epinephrine-activated system (see Fig. 3). In 5 min, phospholipase A_2 hydrolyzed 2.80 μmoles of *l*-α-lecithin. Activation by epinephrine increased the hydrolysis to 7.31 μmoles. This, in turn, was prevented by the addition of 1.0 μg/ml propranolol, and a return to 2.81 μmoles approximated the starting point.

Isoproterenol was also examined. However, the clinical ampoules at our

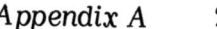

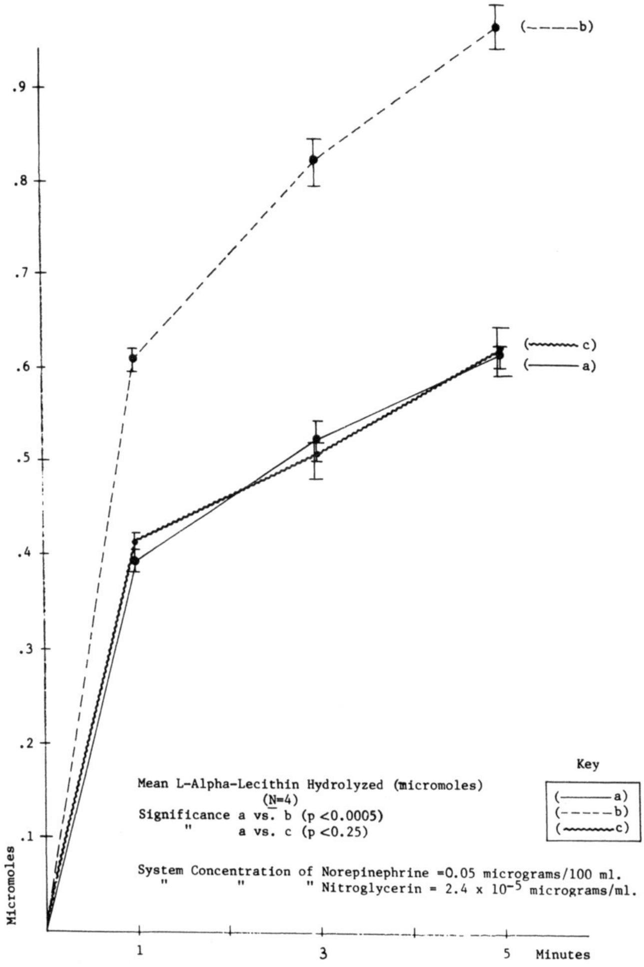

Figure 2. Norepinephrine-activated phospholipase A_2 with nitroglycerin deactivation.

disposal had a diluent which interfered with color development of the reaction. We therefore intend to continue our studies with a plain solution.

DISCUSSION

Our interest in the action of the enzyme phospholipase A_2 was aroused during research on the cause of plasmalogen depletion observed in early atherosclerotic

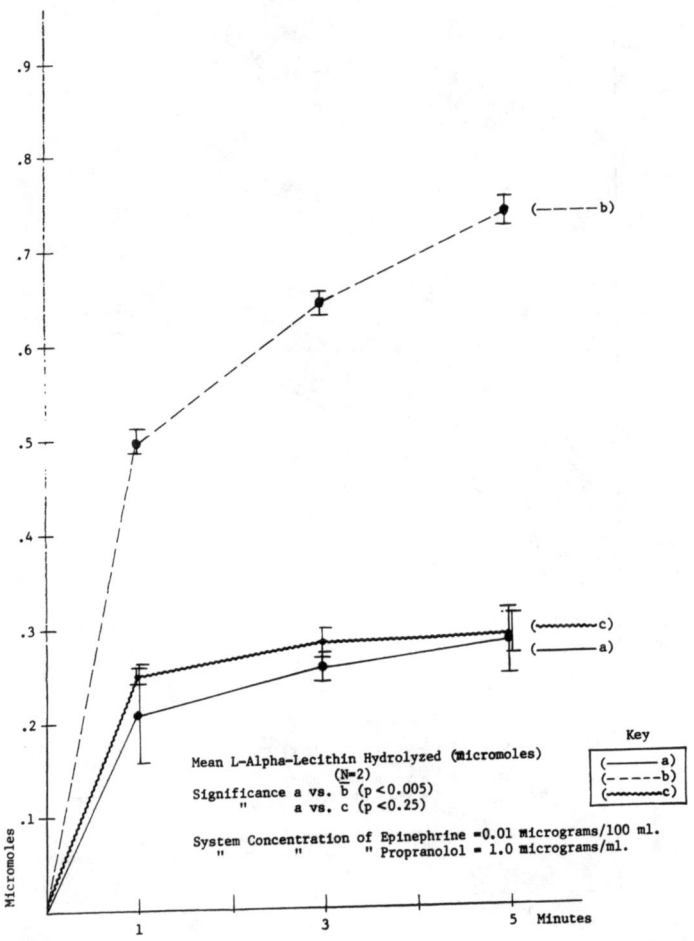

Figure 3. Epinephrine-activated phospholipase A₂ with propranolol deactivation.

lesions and prenecrotic myocardial infarction. The presence of xanthine oxidase in these locations was described (Ross, Ptaszynski, and Oster, 1973). Xanthine oxidase can act on the aldehydic moiety of plasmalogen only if there is first a cleavage of the fatty acid from the ester bond. Phospholipase A₂ seems to require the presence of only one fatty ester linkage adjacent to the alcohol-phosphate bond, and the carbon atom to which this fatty acid is attached must have a precise stereochemical configuration (Gurr and James, 1971).

In a previous publication, it was hypothesized that the known algesic effect of bee venom might be due to its high content of phospholipases, in addition to the presence of polypeptides, apamine, and mellitin (Oster, 1968). One might explain the nature of the pain-producing mechanism by assuming that algesia is caused by: a) the enzyme itself, b) a product of the enzyme action, c) a lack of enzyme substrate, or d) a possible activator of the enzyme. Phospholipases have been found in myocardial cells, either in mitochondria or in lysosomes. We have postulated that the pain experienced in angina pectoris might be associated with the presence of phospholipase A_2 in the myocardium and its algesic activity via one of the four suggested pathways. Use was made of the known pharmacological action of nitroglycerin, i.e., that of possibly aborting attacks of chest pain when administered sublingually. A direct influence of nitroglycerin on the enzyme itself was not found.

It is known that the onset of chest pain is a crescendo phenomenon; i.e., pain is not produced immediately following physical activity or emotional upheaval, but it does occur some time later. We concluded, therefore, that the activation of an eventual pain mechanism could not be a simple pain threshold diminution but, rather, a slow stimulation of a pain-producing metabolic process, which should be influenced by nitroglycerin and/or propranolol in dosages equivalent to those found to be effective *in vivo*. These postulates have found an explanation in our model system.

Oliver (1972) reviewed the evidence supporting local release of catecholamines in the myocardium triggered by ischemia. We have examined the influence of certain biogenic amines on an enzyme situated in the myocardial cell and found a gradual activation of phospholipase A_2 by epinephrine at an optimum 5-min contact with the lecithin substrate and a specific inhibition of this activation by both nitroglycerin and propranolol when added to the enzyme itself. It is of great interest and scientific relevance that this activation of enzyme (phospholipase A_2) by hormone (epinephrine) took place in a cell-free medium without the messenger action of cyclic AMP. This direct action, if paralleled *in vivo*, might have physiological significance for the understanding of other hormone action on cellular enzymes.

The split products of phosphatidyl choline, either a fatty acid (unsaturated or saturated) and/or lysolecithin, display individual pharmacological qualities. Cardiac dysrhythmia has been ascribed to the release of fatty acids from fat depots through lipolysis by catecholamine activation of cyclic AMP. We offer as an explanation the concept of fatty acids released by catecholamine activation of phospholipase A_2 acting on phospholipids. We believe that since fatty acids liberated in such a way are present *in status nascens,* not bound to a carrier protein, their dysrhythmic effect is more direct than that of fatty acids carried in the blood stream from remote reservoirs (Opie, 1972).

Lysolecithins are very active pharmacologically, releasing potassium, inorganic phosphates, and soluble enzymes from muscle cells. The mechanism of action of these substances lies in their detergent qualities, which render the cell membrane more permeable, creating a difference in permeability for many electrolytes (Khairallah and Page, 1960).

Although this study has not yet fully explained what causes the actual pain of angina pectoris, we have created a model which is easily applied to further studies and to investigational manipulation *in vitro* applied to situations which might parallel the *in vivo* condition without interference from extraneous influences.

The fact that lysoplasmalogen exerts a much lesser detergent effect on the cell membrane than lysolecithin (Piantadosi and Snyder, 1970) is considered by us as further confirmation of the prenecrotic plasmalogen depletion concept. When plasmalogen is depleted by the influence of ectopic xanthine oxidase from bovine milk, this protective influence of lysoplasmalogen becomes dissipated. Lysolecithin, arising from the catecholamine activation of phospholipase A_2, can then exert its full detergent force on the cell membrane. This observation is in excellent agreement with previously predicted pathways.

The newly acquired knowledge about the activation of phospholipase A_2 by catecholamine and the influences of nitroglycerin and propranolol have been incorporated into a revised scheme of plasmalogen metabolism (Fig. 4).

Acknowledgment   The authors acknowledge with gratitude the technical assistance of Mr. S. Delco.

REFERENCES

DAWSON, R. M. C. 1963. On the mechanism of action of phospholipase A. Biochem. J. 88: 114.

GURR, M. I., and A. T. JAMES. 1971. Lipid Biochemistry, pp. 140–141. Cornell University Press, Ithaca.

KHAIRALLAH, P. A., and I. H. PAGE. 1960. A vasopressor lipid in incubated plasma. Am. J. Physiol. 199(2): 341–345.

MAGEE, W. L., and R. H. S. THOMPSON. 1960. The estimation of phospholipase A activity in aqueous systems. Biochem. J. 77: 526–534.

MELDRUM, B. S. 1965. The actions of snake venoms on nerve and muscle. The pharmacology of phospholipase A and of polypeptide toxins. Pharmacol. Rev. 17: 393–445.

OLIVER, M. F. 1972. Metabolic response during impending myocardial infarction. II. Clinical implications. Circulation 45: 491–500.

OPIE, L. H. 1972. Metabolic response during impending myocardial infarction. I. Relevance of studies of glucose and fatty acid metabolism in animals. Circulation 45: 483–490.

OSTER, K. A. 1968. Treatment of angina pectoris. Cardiol. Digest (original article) 3: 29–34.

OSTER, K. A. 1972. Role of plasmalogen in heart disease. *In* E. Bajusz and G. Rona (eds.), Recent Advances in Studies on Cardiac Structure and Metabolism, Vol. 1: Myocardiology, pp. 803–813. University Park Press, Baltimore.

PIANTADOSI, C., and F. SNYDER. 1970. Plasmalogens and related derivatives: their chemistry and metabolism. J. Pharmacol. Sci. 59: 283–297.

ROSS, D. J., M. PTASZYNSKI, and K. A. OSTER. 1973. The presence of ectopic xanthine oxidase in atherosclerotic plaques and myocardial tissues. Proc. Soc. Exp. Biol. Med. 144: 523–526.

Liposomes as a Proposed Vehicle for the Persorption of Bovine Xanthine Oxidase (40736)

DONALD J. ROSS, STEPHEN V. SHARNICK[1,2] AND KURT A. OSTER

Department of Biology, Fairfield University, Fairfield, Connecticut 06430

Oster and Mulinos (1) demonstrated the depleting action of bovine milk xanthine oxidase (BMXO) (EC 1.2.3.2) on tissue plasmalogens which are phosphoglyceride analogs of the alkyl-ether acylglycerols. Subsequently, Buddecke (2) demonstrated a definite diminution of plasmalogen in the atherosclerotic plaques of human autopsy material. Similar plasmalogen depletion was found in human myocardial tissue in a case of nonnecrotic myocardial infarction (3). Since plasmalogens constitute 30% of the phospholipids of the human myocardium, Oster hypothesized that such a plasmalogen depletion could initiate a pathological chain reaction leading to cell membrane damage in plasmalogen-rich cardiovascular and nerve tissue (4). Because of the importance that various epidemiological studies (5) ascribe to a dietary cause for atherosclerotic diseases, Oster suggested the possibility that BMXO could represent one such dietary factor in atherogenesis. Experimental evidence for this hypothesis was provided by the discovery of xanthine oxidase in both atherosclerotic plaques and pathological myocardial tissues of human autopsy specimens but not in a normal cardiovascular tissue from the same source (6). Others have demonstrated the absence of xanthine oxidase in normal plasmalogen-rich tissues (7).

That BMXO could be absorbed from the gut, despite its high molecular weight (290,000), is suggested by the presence of serum antibody titers to BMXO in clinically confirmed atherosclerosis patients, as well as in a few "normal" individuals who consumed large amounts of milk (8). The contention of absorption of xanthine oxidase from the gut is further supported in a study in which a population, apparently free of atherosclerotic disease, also showed a range of serum antibody titers to BMXO (9). This work was an extension of Davies' observation that bovine milk antibody titers are significantly increased in the serum of male patients with ischemic heart disease (10).

Although it has been frequently argued that macromolecules are not absorbed by the gastrointestinal tract, it has recently been demonstrated that such molecules as IgG immunoglobulins (MW 188,000) contained in liposomes could enter a cell (11). Liposomes are tiny membranous vesicles formed from various combinations of lipids resembling those found in natural cell membranes. Weissman has demonstrated that liposomes may be formed so as to encapsulate enzymatically active proteins or other macromolecules. Moreover, he has shown that *in vitro* and *in vivo* administration of enzymes by means of liposomes increases the uptake of the liposomes by cellular lysosomes (12). Accordingly, we postulated that the homogenization of whole milk would generate digestion-resistant liposomes with characteristics suitable for transporting BMXO through the intestinal mucosa with eventual deposition on target cell membranes.

Bailie and Morton (13) isolated a milk fraction high in xanthine oxidase activity which was subsequently shown by Hayashi and Smith (14) to possess a high phospholipid-to-protein ratio similar to that found in experimentally generated liposomes. We adapted the procedure of Hayashi and Smith for isolating milk lipoproteins to obtain a fraction from both raw

---

[1] Supported in part by a research grant from the Greater Bridgeport Chapter of the American Heart Association

[2] Present address: University of Connecticut Medical School, Farmington, Conn. 06032.

0037-9727/80/010141-05$01.00/0

and homogenized, pasteurized milk that satisfied the criteria for a liposome, viz., (i) vesicular structure; (ii) isolation through a Sephadex column; (iii) release of the contents of the isolated liposomes by a surface-active agent.

Materials and Methods. Xanthine oxidase assays were performed with a Gilson Differential Respirometer, using the method of Ball (15). Enzyme activity was expressed as microliters of O_2 consumed per milliliter sample per minute at 20°C. The reaction mixture consisted of 1 ml of a $5 \times 10^{-3} M$ xanthine solution, 2 ml of a $0.2 M$ phosphate buffer, pH 7.4, and 2 ml of fraction sample obtained during the purification procedure. Readings, taken at 2-min intervals for 20 min, exhibited a linear relationship between O_2 consumption and time.

The fractionation procedure for both fresh, raw (control), and commercial homogenized, pasteurized cow's milk is outlined in Fig. 1. One part of a stock solution of 10% (w/v) sodium deoxycholate in $0.25 M$ sucrose buffered at pH 8.5 with $0.25 M$ Tris–chloride was added to 9 parts of a pooled commercial whole milk sample. The mixture was stirred for 1 hr at 37°C to release water-soluble lipoprotein from the fat membranes. Samples were centrifuged at various speeds and temperatures as indicated, and the supernatant J was passed through a Sephadex column (40 cm length, 2.6 cm i.d.) packed with Sephadex G-100. The eluant employed was $0.2 M$ phosphate buffer, pH 7.4. The resulting eluate contained the purified liposomes. All flotation layers, supernatant J, and pellets obtained during the course of fractionation were assayed for xanthine oxidase activity which was expressed as a percentage of the original whole milk activity. The lipoprotein-releasing surfactants employed were 3% (w/v) solutions of sodium taurocholate and sodium deoxycholate dissolved in a $0.25 M$ sucrose–$0.25 M$ Tris–chloride at pH 8.5.

Visual identification of the vesicular structure of the purified lipoprotein (PLP) fraction was made with an RCA EMU-3H transmission electron microscope at a magnification of 30,000 X. The fraction was negatively stained with a phosphotungstic acid preparation.

Results. The BMXO activity of whole

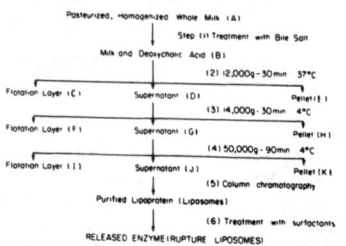

FIG. 1. Isolation and purification procedure for the separation of liposomes from homogenized, pasteurized bovine milk. Whole milk samples were stirred for 1 hr at 25°C in a 1% solution of sodium deoxycholate to release water-soluble lipoprotein from the fat membrane. Centrifugation forces, times, and temperatures are indicated.

milk fractions illustrated in Fig. 1 is reported in Table I as a percentage of the original whole milk sample activity which is assigned a value of 100%. A 70% reduction of activity resulted from both a dilution effect and a partial inhibition of BMXO by the bile salt solution. Small amounts of free enzyme activity accompanied all subsequent fractions. Following the third centrifugation, supernatant J contained 120% whole milk enzyme activity. Approximately a fourfold increase in concentration of water-soluble lipoprotein and free enzyme was found in supernatant J, when compared with xanthine oxidase activity in whole milk treated with bile salt. The lipoprotein component of supernatant J was isolated

TABLE I. BOVINE XANTHINE OXIDASE ACTIVITIES OF THE DIFFERENT FRACTIONS ILLUSTRATED IN FIG. 1 [a]

Fraction	BMXO activity (% of whole milk)
Whole milk (A)	100
Whole milk plus bile salt (B)	30
Pellet (E)	Trace
Flotation layer (C)	3
Pellet (H)	Trace
Flotation layer (F)	Trace
Pellet (K)	Trace
Flotation layer (I)	10
Supernatant (J)	120
Purified lipoprotein (PLP)	8
PLP plus Tween 80	92

[a] Activities of each fraction are expressed as the percentage of the original whole milk activity. Supernatants D and G were not examined for BMXO content because they were preparative fractions.

TABLE II. XANTHINE OXIDASE ACTIVITY OF BOVINE MILK FRACTIONS

Fraction	n [a]	Activity [b] (mean ± SD)	95% C. I. [b,c]
Lipoprotein	15	118 ± 109.7	118 ÷ 61.4
Purified lipoprotein	17	8 ± 4.3	8 ± 2.2
Purified lipoprotein + Tween 80	13	91 ± 46.4	91 ± 28.2

[a] Number of samples.
[b] As percentage of whole milk activity.
[c] 95% confidence interval = $\bar{X} \pm t_{0.05}(\bar{S}_X)$, where $\bar{X}$ = mean sample activity; $t_{0.05}$ = t value at the 0.05 level and for the appropriate number of degrees of freedom; and $\bar{S}_X$ = the standard error of the mean.

from any remaining free enzyme and bile salts by passage through the Sephadex column. Although the final PLP fraction possessed 8% of the original activity, elimination of this residual externally bound enzyme activity can be achieved by a second passage through the column. Addition of either Triton X-100,[3] Tween 80,[3] or both surfactants to the final PLP fraction produced a dramatic increase in BMXO activity which is ascribable to the rupture of the liposomal membrane and subsequent release of the entrapped enzyme (13). Neither of these detergents were found to affect the enzyme activity. Table II shows that the increase in activity was statistically significant ($p \leq 0.05$). An F test showed no significant difference in variance for any of the samples. Commercially pooled milk samples frequently exhibit large variations in their BMXO content. Others have reported similar findings (16).

Two sets of experiments were performed to demonstrate the effects of gastric digestion on the purified liposomes containing BMXO. In the first instance, 100 cc of pasteurized, homogenized milk (pH 6.5) was treated for 2.5 hr at 37°C with 10 cc of artificial gastric juice (pH 1.6) prepared by adding 750 mg of Pepsin USP (Merck) to 100 ml of 0.1 N hydrochloric acid. The resultant mixture, 10:1 (v/v) had a final pH 6. The resulting digest was subsequently subjected to the liposome isolation and purification procedures as outlined in Fig. 1. In the second case, a purified liposomal fraction obtained from pasteurized, homogenized milk was similarly treated (Table III). Significant BMXO activity was retained in both sam-

[3] Obtained from Sigma Chemical Co., St. Louis, Mo.

ples, indicating that the gastric juices failed to completely digest the milk, the PLP, and the liposome-entrapped BMXO.

Figure 2 demonstrates the vesicular structure of the PLP, a morphology characteristic of liposomes. The vesicles range in size from 0.2 to 1 nm. Addition of the surfactants, Triton X-100 or Tween 80, produced the same increase in enzyme activity ascribable to the rupture of the liposomal membrane and subsequent release of the entrapped enzyme (13). Only rare liposomes were observed by electron microscope examination of the raw milk control fractions, and no significant increase in enzyme activity was measurable in these fractions following treatment with the surfactants.

Discussion. An extensive literature on intestinal absorption argues against the possibility that a molecule as large as xanthine oxidase can survive digestion in the stomach and small intestine. However, experimentally produced insulin-containing liposomes, when administered intragastrically, can transport the hormone into the circulation of diabetic rats, lowering the blood sugar (17). Recently, Zikakis *et al.* have shown that BMXO survives the digestive action of the gastrointestinal tract of the rat (18). Ferritin (MW 750,000) can be absorbed from the gut of the adult rat and subsequently detected in various organs but not in blood serum (19). Modern pharmacological studies have repeatedly demonstrated the absorption of liposome-entrapped enzymes, drugs, and other macromolecules. Such liposomal vehicles enhance the bioavailability via the digestive tract of substances which are ordinarily inactivated by this route (20). As far as we know, milk is the only food which, by

TABLE III. XANTHINE OXIDASE CONTENT OF PURIFIED LIPOPROTEIN (PLP) EXPOSED TO GASTRIC JUICE (GJ)

Fraction + GJ	n [a]	Activity [b] (mean ± SD)	95% C. I. [b,c]
Whole milk			
Purified lipoprotein	4	7 ± 0.21	7 ± 0.35
Purified lipoprotein + Tween 80	4	54 ± 3.2	54 ± 5.4
Isolated PLP			
Purified lipoprotein	3	13 ± 0.4	13 ± 1.0
Purified lipoprotein + Tween 80	3	27 ± 1.35	27 ± 2.7

[a] Number of samples.
[b] As percentage of whole milk activity.
[c] 95% confidence interval = $\bar{X} \pm t_{0.05} (\bar{S}_X)$, where X = mean sample activity; $t_{0.05}$ = t value at the 0.05 level and for the appropriate number of degrees of freedom; and $\bar{S}_X$ = the standard error of the mean.

homogenization, artifactually creates enzymes in liposomal form capable of being persorbed by the intestinal mucosa.

In contrast to homogenized, pasteurized milk, raw milk contained only minute amounts of liposomes as demonstrated by measurement of enzyme activity and electron micrographic visualization.

Poste *et al.* conclude that since liposomes are incorporated into the cells as intact structures, their uptake must occur either by endocytosis or by fusion with the cel-

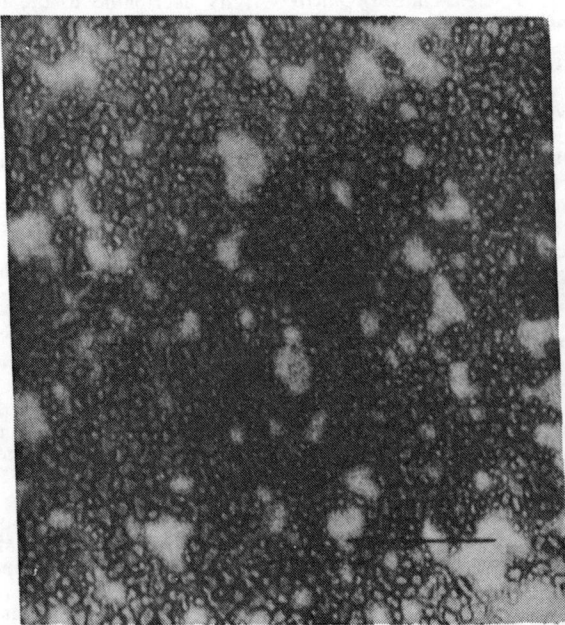

FIG. 2. Electron micrograph of a phosphotungstic acid preparation of the purified liposome fraction of bovine homogenized milk. The scale bar represents 5 μm. (Photographs by Dr. M. Somers, Department of Biology, University of Bridgeport, Bridgeport, Conn.)

lular plasma membrane or both (21). With this suggestion in mind, we looked for BMXO in the particulate structure of human blood. Preliminary milk-loading experiments conducted in our laboratory have indicated that habitual milk drinkers do indeed absorb liposome-bearing BMXO. The enzyme was detectable in the leukocyte fraction of the blood 2 hr after ingestion of 1 liter of homogenized, pasteurized milk. No xanthine oxidase activity was detected in the serum. This is consistent with the observation by others that liposome-entrapped enzymes can be incorporated into other cells (22, 23). Perhaps there is some similarity here to the aforementioned case of ferritin absorption (19). Furthermore, absorption and targeted deposit of milk liposomes can be facilitated by the presence of immune globulins which normally accompany them in mammalian milk (23, 24).

Summary. We present experimental evidence for the hypothesis that bovine milk xanthine oxidase (BMXO) is entrapped in liposomal form by the milk homogenization process. In this form, it will resist gastric digestion and become biologically available. This is the first demonstration of the presence of a liposome-sequestered enzyme in a widely consumed food. The results indicate that a major physical alteration by a technological manipulation of a basic food may have far-reaching biological significance.

1. Oster, K. A., and Mulinos, M. J., Pharmacol. Exp. Ther. 80, 132 (1944).
2. Buddecke, E., and Andresen, G., Hoppe-Seyler's Z. Physiol. Chem. 314, 38 (1959).
3. Oster, K. A., and Hope-Ross, P., Amer. J. Cardiol. 17, 83 (1966).
4. Oster, K. A., Amer. J. Clin. Res. 2, 30 (1971).
5. Stamler, J., et al., Circulation 42, A-55 (1970).
6. Ross, D. J., Ptaszynski, M., and Oster, K. A., Proc. Soc. Exp. Biol. Med. 144, 523 (1973).
7. Morgan, E. J., Biochem. J. 161, 1280 (1926).
8. Rzucidlo, S. J., and Zikakis, J. P., Proc. Soc. Exp. Biol. Med. 160, 477 (1979).
9. Oster, K. A., Oster, J. B., and Ross, D. J., Amer. Lab., Aug., 41 (1974).
10. Davies, D. F., Davies, J. R., and Richards, M. A., J. Athero. Res. 9, 103 (1969).
11. Gregoriadis, G., and Neerunjun, E., Biochem. Biophys. Res. Commun. 65, 537 (1975).
12. Weissman, G., et al. Ann N. Y. Acad. Sci. 308, 235 (1978).
13. Bailie, M. J., and Morton, R. K., Biochem. J. 69, 35 (1958).
14. Hayashi, S., and Smith, L. M., Biochemistry 4, 2550 (1965).
15. Ball, E. G., J. Biol. Chem. 128, 51 (1939).
16. Cerbulis, J., and Farrell, H. M., Jr., J. Dairy Sci. 60, 170 (1977).
17. Dapergolas, G., and Gregoriadis, G., Lancet 2, 824 (1976); Biochem. Soc. Trans. 5, 1383 (1977).
18. Zikakis, J. P., Rzucidlo, S. J., and Biasotto, N. O., J. Dairy Sci. 60, 533 (1977).
19. Hemmings, W. A. (ed.), "Antigen Absorption by the Gut," Chap. 6, p. 49, MTP, Lancaster, England (1978).
20. Gregoriadis, G., N Engl. J. Med. 295, 704 (1976).
21. Poste, G., Papahadjopoulos, D., and Vail, W. J., in "Methods in Cell Biology" (D. M. Prescott, ed.), Vol. 14, p. 33, Academic Press, New York (1976).
22. Weissman, G., Hospital Prac., Sept., 49 (1976).
23. Weissman, G., et al., Proc. Nat. Acad. Sci. USA 72, 88 (1975).
24. Webb, B. H., Johnson, A. H., and Alford, J. A. (eds.), "Fundamentals of Dairy Chemistry," 2nd ed. Avi, Westport, Conn. (1974).

Received April 2, 1979, P.S.E.B.M. 1980, Vol. 163

Kurt A. Oster

Reflections on a Dietary Cause of Atherosclerosis and on its Opponents

When an archaeologist attempts to restore structures of earlier times, his main concern is finding the cause of the destruction of the underlying formations and to rebuild those original forms. He is aided in this enterprise by the discovery of bits and pieces of the structures, shards, coins, and other artifacts. He is less interested in the origin or composition of the superficial layers of dust and debris which, over the centuries, have accumulated and have shielded the underlying relics from discovery.

An analogy can be made with the lesions of atherosclerosis. For the past thirty years, research has been concerned with the origin of the covering of the original injury to the arterial wall. Most researchers have an unhealthy preoccupation with the deposited layers of cholesterol, fibrin, and calcium. They postulate that by lowering serum cholesterol, one not only prevents further deposition of cholesterol but also removes that which is already present, and that by removing these manifestations of the natural healing process, one might then remedy the consequences of the original injury. This approach has not effected greater cardiovascular health, despite the expenditure of billions of scarce research dollars.

I have been seeking to identify a dietary component as the cause of the original atherosclerotic injury to the arterial endothelium and to the heart muscle. Rachel Carson describes in her book, *Silent Spring*, how she noticed the absence of robins. She attributed that observed absence to the toxic effect of an insecticide, DDT. Similarly, I noticed the lack of plasmalogen, a phospholipid, in the early atherosclerotic lesion of the arterial wall and the myocardium and asked the question, "What causes this disappearance?" [1,2]

In order to understand the development of any pathological reaction, one should have a solid knowledge of the original basic stuctures. Without this information, scientific endeavor will degenerate to investigations of association, of circumstantial evidence leading to speculations and exercises in numerology which are given the impressive name of "risk factors". (Someone enumerated 246 of them.[3])

Phospholipids, triglycerides, and lipoproteins, the latter of which also carry cholesterol, are the three main routes of fat transport in humans. Unfortunately, a frequently quoted research paper[4] ascribed to phospholipids the role of "detergents" in human serum. As documentation for this opinion, these researchers rely on their "intuition"[4] but quote no scientific evidence, thereby distorting the equilibrium of scientific inquiry, as one might eliminate one leg from a balanced tripod. Unfortunately, this lopsided approach has dominated most research in atherosclerosis.

Mammalian lipid membranes are composed mainly of phospholipids and cholesterol. The ratio of phospholipids to cholesterol is usually fixed, but in certain pathological conditions, this ratio is changed in favour of an increase in cholesterol over phospholipids. This change of ratio may occur in two ways: (a) an increase in cholesterol in the membrane equilibrium, or (b) a decrease in phospolipids. Both shifts would create disturbances of the sodium pump mechanism and disequilibrate the sodium-potassium flux. Cholesterol is a steroid that modulates the fluidity of eucaryotic membranes.

Ghandi and Ahuja[5] have demonstrated that xanthine oxidase administered intravenously to rabbits oxidized plasmalogen in the heart muscle causing a loss from 10.2 to 2.5% of total lipids, and xanthine oxidase fed as milk fat globules to rats diminished heart plasmalogen from 8.5 to 5.1% of total lipids. The preoccupation with the cholesterol moiety of the cell membrane ignores completely the phospholipid changes. This politically inspired imblance of priorities has let the research of atherosclerosis into a dead-end street.

Plasmalogens may serve as receptors for certain biogenic amines,[6] also, they may be destroyed by the oxidative influence of xanthine oxidase.[7] Findings by us and by others confirmed in human autopsy material that plasmalogens were missing from their usual sites in cases of fresh myocardial infarction without necrosis and in incipient arteriosclerotic lesions (fatty streaks).[2,1,8] These major findings of human pathological histochemistry led to the recognition of a new disease entity which was called "plasmalogen disease"[1] of which arteriosclerosis and myocardial injury may be clinical expressions.

Of great importance is the observation that arterial injury and myocardial injury may occur *simultaneously* and are not necessarily sequelae of the ischemia produced by atherosclerotic plaque obstruction. This observation may explain the occurence of many cardiac arrhythmias without accompanying atherosclerosis.

Since xanthine oxidase is not a constitutive or inducible enzyme in those tissues (except liver) which normally contain plasmalogen in their plasmamembranes, it can be deduced that it is absent from cardiovascular and nerve tissue under ordinary circumstances. This was verified by Morgan in 1926[9] who did an inventory of xanthine oxidase in vertebrate tissues. Oster and Mulinos demonstrated plasmalogen oxidation by topically applying bovine milk xanthine oxidase to guinea pig kidney slices.[7] When the presence of xanthine oxidase was identified in atherosclerotic lesions and myocardial scars, for the first time, this represented the eagerly sought potential cause for the disappearance of plasmalogen from other anatomical locations.[10]

Now what was needed was a dietary source for this ectopic enzyme. I postulated that cow's milk with its very high xanthine oxidase content (120—180 mg) was a possible culprit. Human milk, in contrast, contains only minimum quantities of xanthine oxidase.[11] World-wide studies of milk consumption and death rates from atherosclerotic diseases convinced me that it was not the cow's milk per se but rather the *biological availability* of the xanthine oxidase enzyme so plentifully found in bovine milk that figures so prominently in the pathogenesis of atherosclerotic diseases. Wherever cow's milk was consumed in a boiled or curdled form, the cardiovascular damaging effects were far less evident than the high rates of cardiovascular injury in those areas where milk was consumed as a homogenized product.

An interesting parallel was found in the often witnessed phenomenon of micronized or ultramicronized drugs exerting the same therapeutic results in much smaller dosages than the identical substance administered in macrocrystalline form. Applying sound pharmacological principles to nutrition, the biological availability of "micronized" xanthine oxidase was enhanced by its presence in liposomal entities, which were the end products of the homogenization process.

For the first time, human experiments demonstrated that bovine xanthine oxidase could be carried by white blood cells and not by serum proteins to target organs following consumption of homogenized milk.[12] It also was found that atherosclerotic individuals exhibited unusually high degrees of specific serum antibodies to bovine xanthine oxidase. A suitable test for this determination was devised, using agglutination of tanned sheep red cells.[13] In addition, a therapy against the ongoing destructive influence of xanthine oxidase was discovered in the administration of high doses of a physiological inhibitor, folic acid.[14, 15]

Unfortunately, this logical concept has many detractors, some parochial investigative principles. Objections were raised by National Institutes of Health researchers. D.S. Fredrickson wrote in a letter, quoting outdated text books of physiology, that xanthine oxidase ingested in milk would be destroyed by gastric acidity and intestinal enzymes and that its large molecular size would preclude its passage through the intestinal barrier. These objections were echoed by researchers sponsored by the dairy industry. They neglected to consider that bovine xan-

thine oxidase is consumed in liquid milk, and that milk is an excellent buffer for gastric acidity. Furthermore, the homogenization process creates new physical entities, called "liposomes", which enable most of the protein thus encapsulated to be carried through gastric juices and pancreatic enzymes and remain undigested. A good example for this protective influence is shown in the intestinal absorption of insulin contained in liposomes.[16]

Another objection made by McCarthy and Long,[17] who were able to determine the presence of xanthine oxidase in the serum of 25 "normal" volunteers. They found amazingly unstable enzyme activity, ranging from 0 to 34.6 IU/dl, in contrast to 2,000 "normal" volunteers examined by Al-Khalidi[18] who found zero xanthine oxidase activity. McCarthy and Long also found no xanthine oxidase activity in the serum of milk-fed pigs, implying that the enzyme was not absorbed, but Clark et al[19] reported that feeding a mixture of milk and cream to rats increased their circulating serum xanthine oxidase activity. In contrast to these authors, we could not demonstrate any xanthine oxidase activity in normal human serum either before or after milk consumption, because subsequently we discovered the enzyme sequestered in liposomal form following milk consumption.

The simplistic idea offered first by Fredrickson, that ingestion of xanthine oxidase in homogenized milk should lead to its demonstrable presence in human serum and that its absence from serum is proof of its non-absorption, is, biologically speaking, both naive and untenable. Any absorbed circulating xanthine oxidase would be destroyed by passage of the blood through the liver filter. The reticuloendothelium is the body's well-known protection against introduction of foreign proteins into the system. However, if the foreign protein were present in liposomal form, a different situation would result.

These artificially created vesicles attach themselves to, or are ingested into, white blood cells and can be chemically demonstrated there. This affinity for white blood cells is how liposomes avoid destruction by liver reticulocytes and how liposomal content, such as xanthine oxidase, may be carried to target organs, as the arterial walls and heart muscle, and deposited there. Once ensconced in a foreign or ectopic location, the enzyme exerts its action on the membranes of the cells surrounding it.[12]

Xanthine oxidase will specifically destroy plasmalogen contained in the cell membrane, most probably by the creation of superoxides which are not vulnerable to the influence of serum superoxide dismutase. As a result, the cells so affected can react to this membrane damage by proliferation and eventual necrosis. Thus is created a primary injury which can be repaired according to local conditions. Repair of damage to arterial structures is mostly accomplished by introduction and deposition of cholesterol esters, fibrin, and disintegration material of thrombocytes; injury of the myocardium heals with connective scar tissue formation. Most of these biologically integrated processes may have quite different composition ratios and may feed on themselves after being first established. They may also show some healing tendencies.

These intricate biological findings have been ingnored by the National Dairy Council sponsored work of Ho and Clifford in Davis, California.[20] These researchers failed to consider the difference between the antigenicity of injected and orally administered proteins. They assumed that because xanthine oxidase administered parenterally did not create an atherosclerotic lesion in 13 weeks, the xanthine oxidase theory was thereby disproven, not admitting that the observed diminution of plasmalogen, from 271 to 36 mg, in the myocardium of rabbits was in complete agreement with our findings.

In contrast to Ghandi and Ahuja,[5] Ho and Clifford[21] were unable to determine intravenously administered xanthine oxidase in the myocardium of rabbits. They also claim that xanthine oxidase administration did not deplete the heart or aorta of plasmalogen, again contradicting the results of Ghandi and Ahuja. An examination of the reported results of Ho and Clifford leaves their methodology and conclusion open to serious doubt because of the small number of animals employed in each experimental category (average three or less) and the wide variations of the standard errors; e.g., cholesterol controls of 215 mg/100 G with a standard error of ± 175 mg in three specimens! It is rather difficult to comprehend how the potpourri of conflicting data was permitted to be published in a peer-reviewed journal, even if it satisfied the scientific criteria of Professor Renner.[22] Another inept attempt to criticize the BMXO concept was the inappropriate methodology (everted gut) by Volp & Lage[23] to exclude persorption of a large protein molecule. The method was never designed to attack this problem.

McCarthy's objection to the xanthine oxidase theory[17] also noted in an editorial by members of the American Heart Association Committee on Nutrition,[24] was the so-called non-specificity of the hemagglutination process to detect antibodies against bovine xanthine oxidase and their relation to atherosclerosis. They were referring to the work of Toivanen et al,[25] who used radio-immune assay methods to measure IgM and IgG antibodies to dried milk protein in the blood serum of Finns. They did not note a difference between the amounts of antibodies detected among asymptomatic controls and antibodies found in the myocardial infarction groups. This work followed the original research of Davies et al,[26] who correlated the presence of antibodies to bovine milk found in human blood serum and the prevalence of coronary heart disease, using the same hemagglutination techniques as Oster, Oster, and Ross.[13]

The logic of these experiments is questionable. No one has said that xanthine oxidase is associated with coronary heart disease alone. What Toivanen[25] did was to determine the pervasive influence of milk protein on a population which consumes large amounts of homogenized milk, the Finns, and antibodies to milk proteins were exhibited by both survey groups, those with coronary heart disease and those without. Meanwhile, Davies, in a personal communication, has admitted that the detection of antibodies should be correlated with atherosclerosis in general and not with myocardial infarction alone. The presence of antibodies to bovine milk xanthine oxidase has been also correlated with dairy food intake by Zikakis and his colleagues.[27]

Bierman and Shank[24] maintain that the plasmal reaction takes place under highly acid in vivo conditions (pH 1), wrongfully ascribing a laboratory histochemical staining methodology to a physiological process. This show of examiner misunderstanding echoes

views expressed earlier by Gotto and Jackson.[28] Another objection to the xanthine oxidase theory centers about the fact that human liver and certain parts of the intestine contain xanthine oxidase and that these reservoirs may be the source of the ectopically found enzyme in our investigation.[24] Again, these objections defy simple logic. Human xanthine oxidase does not create specific antibodies; those are derived from xenobiological proteins. Only certain rare autoimmune diseases are ascribed to autoantigenicity of the body's own proteins, like thyroiditis. Al-Khalidi[18] found circulating human xanthine oxidase only in patients with liver disease. Then, if the xanthine oxidase found in human arterial wall lesions would be of human origin, we would have to conclude that atherosclerosis is the result of liver disease. An unlikely assumption, at best.

A JAMA editorial[24] written by the chairman of the American Heart Association Committee on Nutrition also mistakenly equates my biochemical concept of atherosclerosis with causes of coronary heart disease. Heart disease mortality should never be the only criterion of success or failure in the recognition of a disease process.[29] This absurdity was examined in an editorial in 1980, entitled "Duplicity in a Committee Report on Diet and Coronary Heart Disease", wherein the statements of one of the critics from the JAMA editorial were analyzed and found to be equivocal.[30] Statements claiming "...it is far from established fact that the drinking of homogenized milk contributes to mortality from coronary artery disease through the intestinal absorption of bovine xanthine milk..." appear for the justification of the one-sided promotion of lowering serum cholesterol as the only preventative measure against coronary artery disease with no attention to the atherosclerotic process as it occurs in other branches of the arterial tree. The autors do not seem to understand that coronary artery disease is but one manifestation of the complex of atherosclerotic diseases. Since this is not obvious to them, their criticism should be considered of limited value.

I consider Bierman and Shank's[24] statement that the hypothesis has been stated and restated by a single protagonist as an honorable position, not a detraction. Historic precedence has been set by other scientists who were found to be right *after* the establishment fought them and their positions. Furthermore, most of the objections raised by Bierman and Shank have been overcome by further confirming experimentation,[5,12,27] making the single protagonist issue no longer tenable.

No concept of the dietary genesis of atherosclerosis can rest on epidemiological evidence alone, which has contributed to the most recent confusion about the declining reasons for mortality due to coronary heart disease,[31] wherein it is stated unequivocally that clinical studies "gave no firm evidence that cholesterol lowering is beneficial to man. On the other hand, none of these studies shows that cholesterol lowering does not prevent coronary heart disease.. ". The xanthine oxidase concept approaches the cholesterol question from a biochemical angle, since it cannot be denied that high levels of serum cholesterol in man are *associated* with increased severity of atherosclerotic diseases. Other biological sterols, as the male hormone, androsterol, and vitamin D, are also promoters of

the atherosclerotic process.[32] Many of these substances *stimulate xanthine oxidase activity*. Based on the ectopic deposition of bovine milk xanthine oxidase in target organs, maleness, high serum cholesterol and high vitamin D intake could contribute to early and serious atherosclerosis (note that homogenized milk is usually fortified with vitamin D).

As we have enzyme action promoters, so do we also have chemical inhibitors of xanthine oxidase. One of these is estrogens. This fact alone may explain the difference between the lower incidence of atherosclerosis in premenopausal women who universally consume the same diet as men and usually are more sedentary, facts which are often neglected by the epidemiologists. The xanthine oxidase concept of atherogenesis is thereby again put on a firm biochemical footing in contrast to the vagueness of speculative epidemiological observations of risk factors. How are anti-risk factors, like HDL, related to diet?

A therapy for xanthine oxidase-engendered atherosclerosis was developed from careful study of the pertinent biochemical literature. In 1947, Kalckar reported his observation that folic acid is a potent inhibitor of xanthine oxidase.[33] An attempt was made to administer large doses of this physiological substance to patients with proven atherosclerosis, symptomatology and positive xanthine oxidase antibody reactions. The highest dose administered was 80 mg daily, and a monitored serum level of at least 200 ng/dl had to be maintained. With these preconditions, amelioration of the severity of angina pectoris, claudication, and of threatening gangrene, and possibly prevention of secondary heart attacks were accomplished in more than 200 patients over a period of ten years, with no serious side effects attributable to folic acid. This investigation was extended to asymptomatic persons who exhibited high antibody titer to bovine milk xanthine oxidase and who were thus considered at high risk for the development of further atherosclerosis. These persons were given folic acid prophylactically in an attempt to forestall future complications of plasmalogen disease. Folic acid may also contribute to resynthesis of plasmalogen according to Tietz et al.[34]

The significance and success of therapeutic attempts can be ascertained only with large groups of patients observed by many investigators at various medical centers. The seriousness of the problem and the possibility of a solution which is both biochemically plausible and therapeutically and economically feasible are compelling reasons for a project to be undertaken and examined on a large scale. Openmindedness of the scientific society is a precondition for the spread of this research concept, which may promise greater success than the overworked one of lowering serum cholesterol. This BMXO concept does not hold great economic rewards for the drug industry, and the dairy industry is anguished. However, the profits for the public sector would be tremendous, not only in lives saved and lessened morbidity, but also in the economics of the prevention and treatment of a partly man-made disease.

The bovine milk xanthine oxidase theory (1) is conducive to a prevention approach — avoidance of homogenized milk containing biologically available xanthine oxidase; (2) leads to a diagnostic methodology to determine who is affected — xanthine oxidase antibody determination; and (3) is useful as a basis for therapeutic intervention — pharmacological doses of folic acid.

The malignant influence of continous homogenized milk intake containing biologically available xanthine oxidase, especially in youth, is in my opinion, a greater health evil than smoking cigarettes.

*   *   *   *   *

SUMMARY

The present research in the causes of the primary atherosclerotic lesions neglects to investigate the participation of the phospholipids in the disease process, especially the plasmalogen component of the plasmamembrane. The phospholipids of the human myocardium contain 30% plasmalogen which has been found to be depleted in cases of myocardial infarction in humans and in animal experiments by the injection and/or oral administration of bovine milk xanthine oxidase. The early atherosclerotic lesion does not contain any cholesterol whatsoever but shows depletion of plasmalogen.

It has been fairly well established that most atherosclerotic diseases in humans are of dietary origin. The need for the application of modern pharmacological concepts to diet problems is urgent. In the examination of milk intake with regard to the biological availability of xanthine oxidase, it has been demonstrated that the enzyme is contained in liposomal form and follows the physiological pathways of liposomal absorption enabling larger molecules to be delivered via white blood cells to target organs.

This concept has been criticized by research supported by the milk industry and the American Heart Association. It has been shown that the critiques are sophomoric, ill-informed, and inappropriate. The methodologies used in animal experiments are inadequate and flawed with experimental errors. The milk industry, through a public relations' campaign, has attempted to discredit a well established, well researched, and experimentally proven concept of the initiation of atherosclerosis, its detection, and its treatment to the detriment of the advancement of knowledge, thereby damaging public health.

(References, see page 294)

Journal of IAPM   *The Cholesterol Bias Revisited*   Winter, 1983

COMMENTARY

The Cholesterol Bias Revisited
A Different Approach to a Dietary Cause of Atherosclerosis

Kurt A. Oster, M.D.

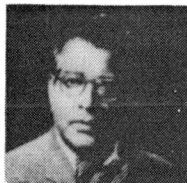

KURT A. OSTER, M.D., Cardiologist and Internist; Emeritus Chairman, Department of Medicine; Emeritus Chief of Cardiology, Park City Hospital, Bridgeport, CT. Dr. Oster is also the Connecticut State Society Representative to the Connecticut Advisory Committee on Food and Drugs. He is a member of the New York Academy of ﹖ences, Society of Experimental Biology and Medicine, Fellow, American College of Cardiology, American Medical Association, Fairfield County Medical Association, Connecticut State Medical Society and Bridgeport Medical Association.

INTRODUCTION

In 1977, during the IAPM Joint Fall Conference in Phoenix, Arizona, I made a presentation which dealt with the "Dietary Goals", expressing doubt about the validity of the concept of dietary goals suggested to the American people by the Select Committee on Nutrition and Human Needs of the U.S. Senate (1977). Also, I questioned some data of the vaunted Framingham Study, which were published in the *Coronary Risk Handbook*, (Insull, 1973) issued by the American Heart Association. A part of my presentation was published in *Connecticut Medicine* (Oster, 1978). Since the controversy about cholesterol-lowering diets continues, the proponents attempt to create a semblance of consensus and a rationale of the diet-heart statement of the American Heart Association. This article will deal briefly with the Eleventh Bethesda Conference Report (1981) and with the AHA Nutrition Committee report (1982).

CONFLICTING REPORTS

I am concerned about the lack of accuracy in some of the data presented at the Eleventh Bethesda Conference by Dr. Jeremiah Stamler (1981). We have been told that individual variations of serum cholesterol cannot be held against the concept of the association of hypercholesterolemia and atherosclerosis. We also have

been told that in order to get a better understanding of this process, we should resort to the comparison of ethnically related groups and their diets. The need for the latter is quite easy to comprehend. However, if one draws conclusions from these groups, one should then quote the findings correctly.

I am baffled by the following discrepancies. Dr. Stamler states (Table XI): "Countries with Decrease or Increase in Rate of Mortality Due to Coronary Heart Disease (men aged 35 to 74 years, 1969 to 1977)," lists Switzerland as having an increase of +7.7%.

Guberan (1979), from the Occupational Health Service of the Canton of Geneva, writes about a surprising *decline* in the cardiovascular mortality in Switzerland from 1951 to 1976, where the mortality was reduced by 30% in males and 40% in females for non-rheumatic heart disease and hypertension. Guberan states, "These reductions were on the whole greater than those observed in the 13 other developed countries studied." He further states, "The 46% fall in milk consumption was balanced by the increasing intake of pork, milk products, and eggs." Thus, contrary to the data obtained for the United States of America (Walker, 1977), the observed trends in cardiovascular mortality are negatively associated with the change in consumption of animal fats and only positively related to milk intake. This latter relationship is in agreement with the surprising association found by Segall (1977) in 43 countries between milk consumption and coronary mortality.

Blackburn (1980), discussing the "Diet-Lipid-Atherosclerosis Relationship: Epidemiological Evidence and Public Health Implication," places Switzerland in the category of those countries which have experienced *no apparent changes* in their CHD death rate from 1968 to 1976.

Referring to WHO's data, TIME magazine, January 12, 1981, page 42, in an article, "A Baffling Coronary Puzzle," lists Switzerland, together with the United States, as a country which has shown a *decrease* of CHD, especially for women. According to Dr. Zbynek Pisa, Chief of WHO's Department of Cardiovascular Diseases, smoking among women and consumption of animal fats are on the upswing.

Stamler lists Sweden also as showing an increase of CHD mortality of +6.9% but, unfortunately, neglects to mention that anti-smoking and other risk reduction campaigns have been vigorously pursued there for many years, demonstrating the futility of his conclusions that we have been on target in undertaking and developing the coronary prevention effort over the last 20 years. The wide gulf between Pisa and Stamler's claims (that the positive changes in life-styles and risk factors among Americans related causally to the decline so far registered in the mortality rates) is evident from the quoted data. Stamler's data are based on the very inaccurate death certificates of coronary heart disease which are of only limited significance. For the unbiased observer, the published data from Stamler, Blackburn, and Pisa appear to be an attempt at hedging their bets and are tailored to individual bias. This does not speak well for the consensus reached in Bethesda.

The Nutrition Committee of the American Heart Association tries to integrate the "best" available evidence on the subject and admits to the high incidence of coronary heart disease in the United States which is in sobering contrast to the glowing reports of CHD death decline. The immense number of costly by-pass operations speaks also against the so far futile and unsuccessful attempts of atherosclerosis prevention recommended by the dietary changes of the AHA. The glaring absence of a pharmacologist in the Nutrition Committee shows the lack of a pharmacologically-based, biological availability concept in reports and research emanating from this Committee. The cautious language that unsaturated fatty acids probably do not possess inherent "toxicity" contradicts the statement of "best" evidence gathered by the Committee.

An unbiased observer may wonder if this "best" evidence is not based on vested interests, deriving both from the justification of enormous sums of previous research money spent and from face-saving attempts to explain the failures and the lack of positive results. Is it not unbecoming for a scientific organization to leave out all contrary results and mention only so-called carefully controlled metabolic studies which are based, in some studies, on the meager number of 12 in a group of individuals (Keys, 1965)?

The doubt about the search for an optimum serum cholesterol was also expressed recently in an article appearing in Lancet (Kannel, 1982) where it is stated: "We must admit to a certain regret that there does seem to be a gradient of CHD risk at low levels of serum cholesterol." The basic policy fault, in my opinion, is that the AHA reports equate CHD with atherosclerosis. This pars pro toto approach will never suffice for the rationality of the search of a dietary cause for cardiovascular lesions and injuries resulting from the ingestion of a food toxin.

HEALTH CARE FUND RAISING

One would expect the American Heart Association to be an open-minded, unprejudiced, scientific body that would scrap any dietary advice they have given to the American people over the years, if it were shown to be incorrect. This organization's funds depend on the generosity of the American public and its expressed desire for a healthy life. However, like many other institutions, it has become instilled with the philosophy, "right or wrong, my association" and will not budge from the stand taken in its pamphlets, cookbook, media jingles, and its teachings of dieticians confused by new approaches. Instead of a science-promoting society, it is in danger of becoming a religion of anticholesterolers who continue to censor opinions different from their own (Oster, 1978).

XANTHINE OXIDASE REVISITED

One should expect that appropriate scientific institutions would welcome, or at least tolerate, varying opinions on major unresolved issues. Yet, the American Heart Association rejected for presentation at its 50th Scientific Sessions a submitted abstract entitled, "Xanthine Oxidase Carrying Liposomes, a Macromolecular 'Trojan Horse' for Atherosclerotic Plaque Initiation."

This is what the American Heart Association did not want to hear. The abstract reads as follows: "One major unresolved problem remains in the genesis of atherosclerosis: What is one of the dietary factors responsible for initiation of the atherosclerotic lesion? Our own studies and those of others have reinforced the contention that xanthine oxidase in homogenized pasteurized bovine milk is absorbed in catalytically active form. Milk liposome-trapped xanthine oxidase can be phagocytized after entering the lymph and thus be released in such target organs as arterial endothelium and the myocardium. Resulting superoxides damage the equilibrium of cell membrane phospholipids by oxidizing plasmalogen, giving rise to smooth muscle cell proliferation, which is the initial lesion. Specific antibodies to bovine xanthine oxidase can be measured in human serum. Large pharmacological doses, 80 mg., of folic acid, a proven xanthine oxidase inhibitor, restores, as a coenzyme, the fatty acid aldehydes needed for plasmalogen synthesis. Applying the 'Trojan Horse' principle of liposomal enzyme passage through the intestinal barrier, a pathway is shown for the initiation of the original atherogenic lesion."

PLASMALOGEN DISEASE

In 1970 I suggested that one of the dietary factors for initiating atherosclerosis was the enzyme xanthine oxidase, ingested and absorbed from homogenized cow's milk. The resultant damage to the tissues of the target organs I called "Plasmalogen Disease," because xanthine oxidase contributed to the degradation of the phospholipid normally referred to as plasmalogen (Oster, 1971). Doubts have been expressed that this large molecule could be absorbed through the human intestine (Carr, 1975). It is my intention to show how recent findings have reinforced my contentions.

MACROMOLECULAR ABSORPTION

Application of modern pharmacological concepts to absorption of foods might easily explain how xanthine oxidase could be an initiating factor in atherosclerosis. I refer now to a recent description of a technique for the introduction of enzymes into lysosomes of enzyme-deficient cells, using immunoglobulin-coated liposomes as carriers for the exogenous enzyme. Introducing a needed enzyme in therapeutic quantities is costly and technically difficult, since the body's immune defenses tend to destroy it rapidly. A "Trojan Horse" is needed to evade immune surveillance (Weisman, 1976).

Liposomes are extremely small particles which can be created artificially from combinations of lipids. The structure of the liposome is onion-like, with many membranes layered concentrically, and the enzyme which was in the original fluid mixture is contained between these concentric layers, forming the liposome.

It is speculated that the use of the principle of trapping substances in liposomal structures may deliver therapeutic modalities to various sites in the body. In actual practice therapeutic substances can be utilized only when suitable immunoglobulins can be incorporated into the exterior liposomal membranes. Aggregation of these immunoglobulins produces a bifunctional ligand which may be phagocytized like a bacterium or a virus, hence the "Trojan Horse" principle.

To release a liposome-entrapped enzyme into the cytoplasm, one needs the addition of 1% lysolecithin to fuse to the liposome without addition of aggregated immunoglobulins. Only 1 to 3% of the enzyme is taken up by this fusion process, in contrast to about 50% by the immunoglobulin-treated liposomes.

This new approach to therapy has been utilized to explain the postulated absorption of xanthine oxidase from homogenized pasteurized bovine milk. In this milieu of micronized liposomes, well examplified by homogenized milk, one finds every ingredient needed to create liposomes with trapped xanthine oxidase. The necessary phospholipids and immunoglobulins are present in abundance. The problem of cell fusion may also be explained by the presence in milk of lysolecithins.

The question arises: can we safely apply the knowledge gained from laboratory-produced liposomes to a food, homogenized milk? According to our latest findings, the answer is yes. The milk fat globule membrane contains 14% lipids, of which 25 to 30% are phospholipids. These phospholipids are mixtures of derivatives of diacylphosphatidic acid, combined with choline, ethanolamine, serines, and inositol.

Sphingomyelins, and, to a lesser extent, cerebrosides and plasmalogen, are also present. One liter of milk contains approximately 120 to 180 mg. of xanthine oxidase, of which at least 50% is catalytically active and biologically available after homogenization and pasteurization (Webb, 1974).

For cytoplasmic fusion, the phospholipids of the milk fat globule membrane contain a small percentage of lysolecithins and lysocephalin. To satisfy the process of diminished antigenicity of liposomal absorption, there is need for immunoglobulins. Bovine milk contains IgG, IgA, and IgM. Instead of the sonication process which was utilized in laboratory experiments with horseradish peroxidase, the homogenization procedure in milk is performed under 2,500 psi, at a speed of 600 to 800 feet per second. The result is reduction of fat globules to about one micron in diameter, a four- to six-fold increase in the fat plasma interfacial surface area. Many of these newly formed fat globules are models for our postulated liposomal structures containing trapped active xanthine oxidase, mostly in monolamellar form (Ross, 1980).

Critics of this concept have argued that ingested xanthine oxidase is destroyed by stomach acidity (Ho, 1976). Arithmetic calculation should convince anyone familiar with the realities of human nutrition that this is not the case. One glass of homogenized milk, 240 cc., can neutralize 1,104 cc. of 0.1 normal hydrochloric acid. Since there are at most only 80 cc. of gastric juice in the empty stomach, or 20 cc. of 0.1 normal hydrochloric acid, one glass of milk would buffer the stomach contents to an almost neutral pH, leaving 75 to 90% of the ingested xanthine oxidase intact. The intestinal proteolytic enzymes will inactivate another small portion of the xanthine oxidase.

Zikakis (1975) has shown that about 36% of the original enzyme reaches the small intestine of rats. Absorption of the enzyme through the intestinal wall as liposomal structures is easily accomplished, and the liposomes reach the arterial blood by way of the lymph.

It would be futile to search for the enzyme in venous blood plasma, as some workers have done. The liposomes in plasma are quickly inactivated by components of the reticulo-endothelial system in the liver and the spleen. Biologically effective liposomes containing the enzyme xanthine oxidase are either phagocytized in lysosomal structures and attack suitable substrates, or they are fused into the cytoplasm of myocardial cells or smooth muscle cells. There they can metabolize plasmalogens of the cell membrane, promoting cell proliferation and many of the other well-described pathological sequelae, depending on the local tissue response. The process of an initial damage to the cell membrane originating from a dietary substance may be accomplished in this way.

Prevention of this pathological process could be accomplished by the creation of a xanthine oxidase-free milk, whose nutritional value would remain unimpaired. The consumer might be given a choice between this milk and the one now available in the market. The 99% fat-free milk approved by the American Heart Association might be termed the "killer milk," because, calorie for calorie, it contains more xanthine oxidase in liposomal structures than its counterpart, the 96.4% fat-free whole milk.

CONCLUSION

In a logical scrutiny of the presented facts, an unbiased observer will conclude that despite vast amounts of money and years of research, the concept that lowering serum cholesterol by diet or drugs will reduce coronary heart disease morbidity and mortality is still unresolved. Therefore, recommendations for dietary changes in the entire American population, based on this concept, should be rejected, at least for the present, as premature, wishful dreams of overzealous workers.

Before we refrain from eating meat, eggs, and dairy products, we must be reasonably certain that the proposed substitutes are wholesome, equally nutritious, and not potentially harmful in the long term. That requires a trial period of at least a generation before judgment can be made.

A proposal is made for the prevention of cell membrane damage by a biologically available ingredient in a food consumed in youth. The concept is based on sound and proven pharmacological principles which, with extended research effort, may well constitute a preventive measure to reduce the incidence of atherosclerotic initiation and concomitant myocardial cell damage.

REFERENCES

American Heart Assn. Nutrition Committee Report, Rationale of the diet-heart statement of the American Heart Assn., Circulation, 65-4:839A-854A, 1982.

Bethesda Conference Report, Am. J. Cardiol., 47-3:713, 1981.

Blackburn, H., Diet-lipid-atherosclerosis relationship: Epidemiological evidence and public health implications. Gotto, Jr., A.M., Smith, L.C., Allen, B., eds. Atherosclerosis V Proceedings of the Fifth International Symposium, Springer-Verlag, NY, 229, 1980.

Carr, C.J., Talbot, J.M., and Fisher, K.D., A Review of the Significance of Bovine Milk Xanthine Oxidase in the Etiology of Atherosclerosis, Life Science Research Office, Bed. Am. Soc. of Exper. Biol., Bethesda, Maryland, 1975.

Diet Related to Killer Diseases II, Hearings before the Select Committee on Nutrition and Human Needs of the U.S. Senate, 95th Congress, February 1 and 2, 1977, U.S. Government Printing Office, Washington, 1977.

Guberan, E., Surprising decline of cardiovascular mortality in Switzerland: 1951-1956. J. Epidemiol. and Community Health, 33:114-20, 1979.

Ho, C.J. and Clifford, A.J., Digestion and absorption of bovine milk xanthine oxidase and its role as an aldehyde oxidase, J. Nutr., 106:1600-1609, 1976.

Insull, Jr. W., Coronary Risk Handbook, based on Framingham Study 16-year follow-up, American Heart Assn., Inc., Dallas, Texas 1973.

Kannel, W.B., Gordon, T., The search for an optimum serum cholesterol, The Lancet, 374-375, Aug. 14, 1982.

Keys, A., Anderson, J.T., Grande, F., Serum cholesterol response to changes in the diet. II. The effect of cholesterol in the diet, Metabolism, 14:759, 1965.

Oster, K.A., Plasmalogen diseases: a new concept of the etiology of the atherosclerotic process, Am. J. Clin. Res., 2:30-35, 1971.

Oster, K.A., Dietary goals — dreams and reality, Conn. Medicine, 42-11:705-708, 1978.

Ross, D.J., Sharnick, S.V., and Oster, K.A., Liposomes as a proposed vehicle for the persorption of bovine xanthine oxidase, Proc. Soc. Exp. Biol. and Med., 163:141-145, January 1980.

Segall, J.J., Is milk a coronary health hazard? Br. J. Preventive and Social Med., 31:81-85, 1977.

Walker, W.J., Changing United States life-style and declining vascular mortality, cause or coincidence, N. Engl. J. Med., 297:163-165, 1977.

Webb, B.H., Johnson, A.H. and Alford, J.A., Fundamentals of Dairy Chemistry, 2nd ed., pp. 572-576, The Avi Publishing Co., Westport, CT., 1974.

Weisman, G., Experimental enzyme replacement in genetic and other disorders, Hosp. Pract., 11:49-58, 1976.

Zikakis, J.P., Rzucidlo, S.J., Biasotto, N.O., Persistence of bovine milk xanthine oxidase activity after gastric digestion, in vivo, in vitro, J. Dairy Sc., 58:1238, 1975.

C●SMETIC
DERMATOLOGY

The Case of the Missing Risk Factor

Kurt A. Oster, MD

Dr. Oster is the internist who has had the temerity to suggest that we Americans suffer more heart attacks than comparable population groups, not because we over-indulge in cholesterol but because we "tinker" with our nutrition and try to improve upon nature. He states that possibly a simple thing like the homogenization of milk has been just enough to unhinge an enzyme system so that noxious lipid plaques are deposited in our arteries rather than being stored as energy fuel. Most cardiologists regard this concept as heretical, yet in all probability the reasoning is absolutely correct.

The following article appears in this column because much of dermatology, particularly that concerned with the physiological ineffectiveness of topically applied agents, has been thwarted by concepts; we too need an imaginative breakthrough. —HERBERT J. SPOOR, MD

More effort now seems to be expended in attempting to eradicate disease "risk factors" than is spent in treating those diseases and discovering and clarifying their causes. We are told that eliminating or diminishing the risk factors will enable us to reduce the incidence of many manifestations of atherosclerosis, chiefly myocardial infarction. The truth of this rather naive attitude in medical therapeutics has never been shown, although one could cite myriad examples in medical history

when this approach to disease control has failed miserably.

During this country's colonial history and even later, "bad blood" was the risk factor associated with many undiagnosed diseases. To eliminate this risk factor people were bled, leeches and cups were applied, skin was scarified. These were therapeutic methods recommended and used by the contemporary medical establishment. Garrison, in his history of medicine wrote: "It took a long time to demonstrate that the advancement of internal medicine as a science can never be accomplished by hugging some pet theory out of regard for its author's personality, but only through the performance of a vast amount of chemical, physical and biological research by thousands of willing workers. The first step in this direction was taken by Broussais, who did away with metaphysical conceptions of disease only to substitute something worse."[1]

At this juncture we find ourselves in a similar situation regarding the prevention and treatment of atherosclerosis by the diminution of a so-called risk factor, serum cholesterol. A thoughtful Swedish clinician, Lars Werko, wrote in 1971: "A current population study indicates that removal of only one risk factor may have little or no impact on the overall morbidity or mortality in middle-aged men in western societies. . . . The hypothesis that removal of several risk factors will decrease the incidence of ischemic heart disease in the community must be tested before any large-scale changes are advocated in our

Reprint requests to the Department of Biology, Fairfield University, Fairfield, Connecticut.

Cosmetic Dermatology (continued)

life style."[2] Yet G. Rose, a British researcher, stated in the same year, "The Americans with their unfortunate excess incidence rate suggest the need to search for some other factor, factor x, which is very uniform for all the American subjects in the study."[3] Keys and his associates, measuring and comparing all known risk factors, have found that a group of Europeans with the same risk factor profile as Americans have 50% fewer heart attacks.[3] Quite a difference for people with the same ethnic backgrounds.

Not enough investigators admit the possibility that the accused may be completely innocent. The recommended lowering of serum cholesterol so persistently advocated by "authorities" and prestigious societies may be the misguided first cousin of the recommendations of Broussais and his pupils who "adopted a powerful antiphlogistic or weakening regime, the main features of which were to deprive the patient of his proper food and to leech him all over his body."[1]

Until we have discovered the true cause of atherosclerosis, especially in youth, we should, as good physicians, be wary of the food faddists and the pragmatists who recommend untried remedies whose risks, known or unknown, may be greater than doing nothing or giving a placebo. Realization of the existence of a near epidemic of heart attacks should not plunge us into apocalyptic despair, clutching at every straw of pseudosolution. Fear has provoked certain false prophets to persuade us to substitute blind faith for cool reason. Let us be candid before we submit to tangential thinking with artificial and unproven recommendations which might just boomerang.

References

1. Garrison FH: An Introduction to the History of Medicine ed 4, pp 408–409, Philadelphia: W. B. Saunders, 1961.

2. Werko L: Can we prevent heart disease? Ann Intern Med 74:278, 1971.

3. Tibblin G et al: Preventive Cardiology, pp 65–72, New York: John Wiley and Sons, 1971.

References.

1. Oster, K.A. Amer. J. Clin. Res. 1971, 2:30–35.

2. Oster, K.A. and Hope-Ross, P. Am. J. Cardiol. 1966, 17:83–85.

3. Hopkins, P.N. and Williams, R.R. Atherosclerosis. 1981, 40:1–52.

4. Fredrickson, D.S., Levy R.I., and Lees R.S. N. Eng. J. Med. 1967. 276:215–226,   273–281.

5. Gandhi, M.P.S. and Ahuja, S.P. Zbl. Vet. Med. 1979. A26–635–642.

6. Oster, K.A. Nature (London). 1942. 50:108.

7. Oster, K.A. and Mulinos, M.G. J. Pharm. Exp. Ther. 1944, 80:132.

8. Buddecke, E. and Andresen, G. Hoppe Seiler's Z. Physiol. Chem. 1959, 314:38.

9. Morgan, E.J. Biochem. J. 1926, 161:1280.

10. Ross, D.J., Ptaszynski, M., and Oster, K.A. Proc. Soc. Exp. Biol. Med. 1973, 144:523–526.

11. Zikakis, J.P., Dougherty, T.M., and Biasotto, N.O. J. Food Sci. 1976, 41:1408–1412.

12. Ross. D.J., Sharnick, S.V., and Oster, K.A. Proc. Soc. Exp. Biol. Med. 1980, 163:141–145.

13. Oster, K.A., Oster, J.B., and Ross, D.J. Am. Laby. 1974, August 41–47.

14. Oster, K.A. Arteriosclerosis i. 1981, Page 1.

15. Oster, K.A. Abstract Federation Proceedings. 1981, 40–3.

16. Gregoriadis. G. N. Eng. J. Med. 1976, 295:704.

17. McCarthy, R.D. and Long, G.A. J. Dairy Sci. 1976, 59:1059–1062.

18. Shamma'a, M.H., Nasrallah, S.M., Al-Khalidi U.A. Am. J. Dig. Dis. 1973, 18:15–22.

19. Clark, A.J., Pratt, D.E., Chambers, J.V. Life Sciences 1976, 19:887–892.

20. Ho, C.Y. and Clifford, A.J. J. Nutr. 1976, 106:1600–1609.

21. Ho, C.Y. and Clifford, A.J. J. Nutr. 1977, 107:758.

22. Renner, Deut. Med. Wochensch. 1979, 104:45.

23. Volp, R.F. and Lage, G.L. Proc. Soc. Exp. Biol. Med. 1977. 154:488.

24. Bierman, E. and Shank, R.E. JAMA. 1975, 234:630–631.

25. Toivanen, A. et al. Lancet 2, 1975, Page 205.

26. Davies, D.F., Davies, J.R., and Richards, M.A. J. Atheroscler. Res. 1969, 9:103:107.

27. Rzucidlo, S.J. and Zikakis, J.P. Proc. Soc. Exp. Biol. Med. 1979, 160:477–482.

28. Gotto, Jr., A.M. and Jackson, R.I. N. Eng. J. Med. 1974, 290–16:913.

29. Detre, K.M., Ware, J., and Mantel, N. Circulation. 1981, 64:667–668.

30. Oster, K.A. Am. Heart J. 1980, 99–4; 409–412.

31. Levy, R.I. Arteriosclerosis I. 1981, Pages 312–326.

32. Roussos, G.G. Biochim. Biophys. Acta. 1963, 73–338.

33. Kalckar, H.M. and Klenow, H. J. Biol. Chem. 1948, 172:349–350.

34. Tietz, A., Lindberg, M., and Kennedy. E.P. J. Biol. Chem. 1964, 239:4081.

The egg controversy: are eggs good or bad?

Dear Sir:

I think that the article in the October 1981 issue of *the American Journal of Clinical Nutrition* by Roberts et al (1) should be critically examined. The authors come to the conclusion that feeding of whole eggs in a double-blind study in outpatients eating their customary diets had a hypercholesterolemic effect compared to a cholesterol-free product. They implied that the hypercholesterolemic effect contributes to an increase of atherosclerosis and heart attacks. They also stated that results of early metabolic experiments are confirmed. This research already has been incorporated as a key reference on diet. One does not doubt that the data presented are factual, but what is very much in question is the relatedness of the present study to other investigations (2–5) which have not found any significant changes in serum cholesterol with the addition of eggs to the home diet of adult men and women.

Also, the addition of two whole eggs to the regular diet of hospitalized patients has not shown any significant increase in serum cholesterol. My own unpublished studies of two hospitalized patients with a daily feeding of two eggs, extending over a period of 2 yr did not produce any serum cholesterol increase whatsoever. There was a minimal increase after the 1st month of 5% which returned to the original level and remained unchanged over the entire period of 2 yr.

One wonders how such variance in results of egg consumption and cholesterol changes could happen, especially since this issue was in the foreground of the Federal Trade Commission trial of the United States government against the National Commission on Egg Nutrition in 1975, in which Connor was a government witness. This discrepancy in scientific reports of finding no changes in serum cholesterol after shell egg consumption on one hand and elevation of serum cholesterol after homogenized egg consumption, on the other hand, needs definite scrutinizing analysis because so much has depended on the wording and the semantics applied in the claims and counterclaims. This letter serves to focus on some of the issues in question.

Connor et al stress the double-blind approach of their experimental protocol. In actuality, it was a triple-blind experiment. They were depending on the manufacturer of the frozen homogenized whole eggs and apparently were unfamiliar with the physical characteristics of the homogenization process, resulting in the end product prepared by Standard Brands, Inc, a commercial firm with monetary interest in promoting the comparative and competitive product (Egg Beaters).

The Connor group does not familiarize the reader with the actual process of homogenization of whole eggs. Are there now new micellae formed which contain cholesterol in a liposomal form? What is the mean particle size of the homogenized product? How much oxidation of cholesterol took place? They provide product composition data, but this is not enough information for serious nutrition research. As Connor himself claims in his discussion of the Tarahumara Indians' studies, it is known that crystalline cholesterol is poorly absorbed in contrast to egg yolk cholesterol (6).

I think there exists an urgent need for nutrition science to follow the example of pharmacology and pharmaceutical product preparation both of which stress the importance of biological availability of a product. Disregarding this concept leads to unexplainable and nonscientific results causing unnecessary controversy. The concept of availability of chemicals is of utmost importance in generic drug research and should be grafted as a branch of scientific nutrition.

Just as homogenization of milk will produce increased bioavailability of an enzyme, xanthine oxidase (7), so will homogenization of an egg increase the biological availability of cholesterol. This was beautifully proven by Thompson et al (8), who stated in 1968: "These findings suggest that mixed micellar lipid increased the rate of appearance of labeled free cholesterol and vitamin D_3 in lymph by enhancing their transport out of the intestinal mucosa, rather than by an effect on uptake." Connor ignores this biological fact and equates homogenized artifacts with the natural product of a shell egg.

Broad (9) quotes a philosopher of science,

The American Journal of Clinical Nutrition 36: DECEMBER 1982.   Printed in USA
© 1982 American Society for Clinical Nutrition

Paul Feyerabend, as saying ". . . that no theory, no matter how good, ever agrees with all the facts in its domain. A scientist must therefore rhetorically nudge certain facts out of the picture, defuse them with an ad hoc hypothesis or just plain ignore them." Also, Thomas S Kuhn was quoted to say "that during normal periods, anomalies observed by the scientist must be suppressed or ignored."

It is also useful to consider a recent editorial on "Science and advertising" (10), which states: "A more pernicious, but less obvious, form of advertising is practiced by the investigator who massages his raw data to eliminate or add results that help to confirm his biases. When wittingly performed, such an excuse is strongly criticized by scientific disciplinarians and occasionally become highly publicized; but the process in a more subliminal form may be more common than we like to admit, probably because of the unique vagaries of biologic data."

I suggest that Connor's equating homogenized eggs with shell eggs is unwarranted and scientifically untenable. It has been adequately shown by respected scientists (2-5) that eating shell eggs in a nonhomogenized form by normal persons will not cause a significant increase in serum cholesterol and therefore constitutes no subsequent greater risk of atherosclerosis and heart disease. It should be reasonably concluded that those who have no cholesterol metabolism problem may continue to eat shell eggs without putting their health in jeopardy.

Kurt A Oster, MD

Adjunct Research Professor
Fairfield University
Department of Biology
Fairfield, CT 06430

References

1. Roberts SL, McMurry MP, Connor WE. Does egg feeding (i.e., dietary cholesterol) affect plasma cholesterol levels in humans? The results of a double-blind study. Am J Clin Nutr 1981;34:2092-9.
2. Slater G, Mead J, Dhopeshwarkar G, Robinson S, Alfin-Slater RB. Plasma cholesterol and triglyceride in men with added eggs in the diet. Nutr Rep Int 1976;14:249-60.
3. Porter MW, Yamanaka W, Carlson S, Flynn M. Effect of dietary egg on human serum cholesterol and triglyceride of human males. Am J Clin Nutr 1977;30:490-5.
4. Flynn MA, Nolph GB, Flynn TC, Kahrs R, Krause G. Effect of dietary egg on human serum cholesterol and triglycerides. Am J Clin Nutr 1979;32:1051-7.
5. Kummerow FA, Kim Y, Hull J, et al. The influence of egg consumption on the serum cholesterol level in human subjects. Am J Clin Nutr 1977;30:664-73.
6. McMurry MP, Connor WE, Cerqueira MT. Dietary cholesterol and the plasma lipids and lipoproteins in the Tarahumara Indians: a people habituated to a low cholesterol diet after weaning. Am J Clin Nutr 1982;35:741-4.
7. Ross DJ, Sharnick SV, Oster KA. Liposomes as a proposed vehicle for the persorption of bovine xanthine oxidase. Proc Soc Exp Biol Med 1980;163:141-5.
8. Thompson GR, Ockner RK, Isselbacher KJ. Effect of mixed micellar lipid on the absorption of cholesterol and vitamin D_1 into lymph. J Clin Invest 1969;48:87-95.
9. Broad WJ. Fraud and the structure of sciences. Science 1981;212:137-41.
10. Cohn JN. Science and advertising. Circulation 1982;65-5:839-40.

Dietary cholesterol and atherosclerosis: the Tarahumara (Flying Feet) Indians

Dear Sir:

The low level of serum cholesterol of the Tarahumara Indians is used extensively in the literature as an example of excellent dietary accomplishment. McGill (1) quotes from studies on the plasma lipids, lipoproteins, and diet of the Tarahumara Indians of Mexico by Connor et al. (2).

The Tarahumara Indians' diet consists primarily of beans, corn, and squash. Their mean male cholesterol level is 136 mg/dl ±27. The average daily intake of cholesterol is 71 mg for adult men; for children, a mere 33 mg/day. Total fat intake is 38 g/day for men and 28 g/day for women, providing 11 to 12% of calories from fat of which only 20% is saturated. Eggs contribute about 70% of dietary cholesterol.

Connor et al. (2) state that "the total plasma cholesterol correlated positively with dietary cholesterol intake (r = 0.874), emphasizing that *the first time in man* such a correlation has been found." They conclude, mentioning the absence of hypertension, obesity, and the usual age rise of serum cholesterol in adults, "*thus the customary diet of the Tarahumara Indians is adequate in all nutrients, is hypolipidemic, and is presumably antiatherogenic*" (emphasis mine).

The cited benefits of low cholesterol, low-fat diets must be evaluated in the overall life context of adults and children. The nub of the "dietary goals" recommendations is distressingly similar to the nutrition of the Tarahumara Indians. One may read between the lines that their diet, allowing a high degree of physical activity and freedom from coronary heart disease, might approach the ideal diet for the combatting of "killer diseases" expounded by Senator McGovern's Select Committee on Nutrition.

My interest in good nutrition was piqued, and though no expert on the mores and habits of the Tarahumara Indians, I sought other sources of information about this tribe, about its lifestyle, its life expectancy, and its social customs. I found suitable information in a completely objective article by the editor of the *National Geographic*, W. E. Garrett (3). This article, accompanied by excellent photographs, gives a neutral observer's findings of the Tarahumaras, a tribe among the most primitive Indians left in North America.

During a week's stay at a Jesuit clinic, Garrett learned that "*80% of the Tarahumaras die before five of malnutrition or disease*" (emphasis mine). Uncertain and reserved in social contact with outsiders, the Tarahumaras live in the shadow of famine despite efforts by Mexico's National Institute of Indian Affairs to improve their lot. They can coax only meager crops from the rocky soil. Though they herd cattle, sheep, and goats and use the manure as fertilizer, they never milk the cows and usually kill animals only for religious feasts."

I believe that the editors of *The American Journal of Clinical Nutrition* should have been provided with this evidence and should have informed its readers that this tribe, which has been quoted as a paragon of nutrition, actually is at the brink of famine and pays a frightful price to keep its plasma cholesterol low. I fear the so-called correlation of its plasma cholesterol value with its dietary cholesterol intake is an expression of the absolute minimum plasma cholesterol may reach before lack of resistance to disease and pathology develop. The low plasma cholesterol values of the Tarahumaras should be considered an aberration of an insufficient diet and not as a norm to be emulated by followers of an unproven hypothesis. The oft reiterated statement that diets which result in a low plasma serum cholesterol will not cause any health damage is again found wanting in one of nature's own experiments.

It certainly speaks poorly for any recommendation to persuade American mothers to give their children a diet aimed at lowering plasma cholesterol values to levels approaching those of the Tarahumara Indians. To purposely neglect to mention in a scientific article about nutrition the eventual side effects—as in this case of high child mortality—is quite irresponsible, in my opinion. Similarly, a drug manufacturer is required to men-

The American Journal of Clinical Nutrition 34: JUNE 1981, pp. 1167–1169. Printed in U.S.A.
© 1981 American Society for Clinical Nutrition

tion observed adverse effects of a drug. Generally speaking, defective scientific information may lead to false conclusions and costly and predictably unsuccessful experimentation, and contribute to the lack of credibility and disrepute of nutritional research.

Lowering of plasma cholesterol might not be the highly propagandized remedy for the prevention and treatment of atherosclerosis. Different approaches to the solution of the problem of this terrible disease are urgently needed.

Addendum

Since this article was written in January 1980, it has been found that recommendations for diets similar to that of the Tarahumara Indians have been widely disseminated. A book on the national bestseller list states that the Pritikin Diet is roughly the equivalent of that of the Tarahumara Indians; 10% protein, 10% fat, and 80% complex carbohydrates. Exceptional athletic feats of some members of the tribe are mentioned as a quasi-testimonial (4).

Also, Blackburn (5) singles out the low total serum cholesterol of the Tarahumaras and calls them "one fascinating 'natural experiment.'" He claims that "the Tarahumaras are almost entirely vegetarian and are among the more active ethnic groups on earth. Also, they are lean and consume considerable amounts of alcohol as fermented corn beer. They do not smoke heavily." They are reported to have one of the lowest high-density lipoprotein values and low high-density lipoprotein/total cholesterol ratios.

Both authors fail to mention the high child mortality and the malnutrition of the tribe (3) in their praise of the Tarahumara Indians' diet.

Kurt A. Oster, M.D.

Adjunct Research Professor
Department of Biology
Fairfield University
Fairfield, Connecticut 06430

References

1. McGill W. The relationship of dietary cholesterol to serum cholesterol concentration and to atherosclerosis in man. Am J Clin Nutr 1979;32(suppl):2664.
2. Connor WE, Cerqueira MT, Connor RW, Wallace RB, Malinow R, Casdorph HR. The plasma lipids, lipoproteins, and diet of the Tarahumara Indians of Mexico. Am J Clin Nutr 1978;31:1131.
3. Garrett WE. South to Mexico City. Natl Geo 1968;134:145.
4. Pritikin N, McGrady PM Jr. The Pritikin program for diet and exercise. New York: Grosset & Dunlap, Inc., 1979.
5. Blackburn H. Diet-lipid-atherosclerosis relationship: Epidemiological evidence and public health implications. In: Atherosclerosis V. Gotto AM Jr, Smith LC, Allen B, eds. New York: Springer-Verlag, 1980: 220.

December 4, 1973

Letters to the Editor
The New York Times
229 West 43rd Street
New York, NY

Dear Sir:

    In her November 29 article, "The Egg Falls Victim to Cholesterol Fears," Jane Brody made some very questionable statements, which is unbecoming to an objective science reporter who should not show bias. The curve accompanying her article shows per capita egg consumption falling from 400 in 1945 to 300 in 1973. These figures give the lie to the American Heart Association stand that cholesterol intake is increasing. Despite decreased egg consumption, reduced milk intake and replacement of butter by margarine, which contains artificial fatty acids, the "epidemic" of heart attacks continues to grow. Every attempt at cholesterol reduction in humans has met with failure as far as reduction of heart attacks is concerned. Even the most fanatical low-fat and low-cholesterol diet faddist would not dare to claim that this diet has been proven to reduce the incidence of heart attacks.

    Who are the "leading authorities" mentioned by Ms. Brody who call the egg industry statements "irresponsible," "inaccurate," and a "gross distortion of the facts?" Physicians in general are notoriously poorly informed about the biochemistry, pharmacology, and immunochemistry involved in the study of nutrition and the utilization of food by human beings. I am vitally interested in research on the causes of atherosclerosis and will gladly defend the egg industry against the threaten-

ed complaint to the Federal Trade Commission
by the Action on Safety and Health organization.
The contention that "there is absolutely no scientific evidence that eating eggs increases the risk
of heart disease" in otherwise healthy people is
100 percent correct.

Dr.William E. Connor may be an authority
on cholesterol toxicity in monkeys, but this feat
cannot be applied to humans. His experiments
show only that monkeys can be poisoned by unnatur-
ally high cholesterol feeding, creating a kind of
storage disease resembling atherosclerosis. Humans
do not eat the proportion of cholesterol Dr. Connor
uses to poison his monkeys. To apply his experiments to the human disease which starts in child-
hood when no large amounts of cholesterol are
consumed is unscientific, unwarranted and futile.

In an earlier article (November 16) Ms. Brody
reported on another misguided attempt to prevent
heart disease, a nutritional scheme in Arizona
to reduce protein, cholesterol and saturated fat
intake in children. She wrote, "(Although) there
is no established proof that such a program will
have the desired effect of preventing premature
death and disability from heart and blood vessel
diseases." Unwittingly she stated almost verbatim
what the National Commission on Egg Nutrition
has been saying all along.

Which Jane Brody is to be believed, the one
from November 16 or from November 29?

Kurt A. Oster, M.D.

Reprinted From

Medical Tribune

August 9 and August 23 1978

Atheroma Sleuth Defends Lipids, Blames Heart Disease on Milk Making

By NATHAN HORWITZ
Medical Tribune Report

BRIDGEPORT. CONN.—Is homogenized pasteurized cow's milk the missing key to the riddle of atherosclerotic disease?

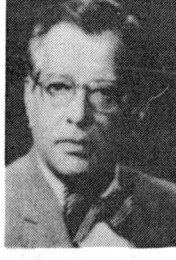

DR. OSTER

Even as the popular lipid hypothesis links atherogenesis to foods ranging from eggs and cheese to marbled beef and avocados, dissenting voices insist it's an unproved concept bristling with unanswered questions. They urge that other, more plausible and biochemically simpler explanations be sought for arterial plaque buildup.

Prominent among the dissenters is Dr. Kurt A. Oster, Emeritus Chief of Cardiology at Park City Hospital here, who proposes what may well be the most developed alternative hypothesis to date. The core of Dr. Oster's admittedly controversial view is that homogenized milk, proud product of a sanitized society, is one of the central atherosclerotic culprits. The process of homogenization itself, Dr. Oster contends, makes possible the release of a milk-borne enzyme—xanthine oxidase (XO)—that triggers the primary atherosclerotic lesion, opening the biochemical pathway to degenerative sequelae.

When this enzyme is biochemically un-available, as in milk-drinking societies that boil but do not homogenize their milk, or in societies that drink little or no cow's milk, Dr. Oster notes that the coronary artery disease rate is low. Two examples: France and India.

The therapeutic corollary of this hypothesis is the clinical discovery that high doses of folic acid, a xanthine oxidase inhibitor, prevents or arrests the progress of dietary atherosclerosis. In a preliminary report on a long-term study of folic acid in some 200 subjects, Dr. Oster noted a "significant" decline in angina pectoris and recurrent myocardial infarction in the treated group, compared with controls.

Dr. Oster, who first proposed his basic concept in 1970 and has since developed it in a series of studies, argues that it bypasses the thicket of puzzles and inconsistencies in the lipid story and offers, for the first time, both a reproducible explanation and the basis for a rational prophylaxis in atherosclerosis. It is, in short, a unitary hypothesis.

Although the 67-year-old scientist's studies have been published in a number of specialty journals, and he has won the support of some researchers, he is an embattled figure, albeit a cheerfully embattled one. The American Heart Association last year refused to accept an abstract of his latest work for publication in the annual meeting program. Recently, one of the nation's most prestigious journals rejected his latest paper after the referee commented that he saw no reason "to give a controversial viewpoint a national forum."

Dr. Oster was grimly amused: "If science has no room for controversy, what does?"

Nevertheless, some major authorities feel Dr. Oster's findings warrant further investigation. In 1975, the Food and Drug Administration commissioned a number of its consultants to prepare a study of the Oster hypothesis. Although the experts reported that the data were, in their view, "inconclusive," they proposed a series of investigations to clarify some of the unanswered problems. **One of their major questions was how a molecule as large as xanthine oxidase is able to leave the gastrointestinal tract to inflict its damage on the arterial endothelium.**

Dr. Oster, who is Adjunct Research Professor of Biology at Fairfield University, reports that current work by himself and his collaborators may have identified the answer to that and thus, possibly, completed the theoretical structure of his hypothesis.

In his model of diet-induced atherosclerotic lesions, xanthine oxidase in homogenized bovine milk is absorbed from the intestinal tract, circulates, and is deposited in catalytically active form in the tissues of the target organs—the myocardium and arterial endothelium. Here it reacts with plasmalogen, a phospholipid fraction of cell membranes, to initiate smooth muscle proliferation, the primary lesion of atherosclerosis. **Subsequent cholesterol infiltration and fibrin build-up in the endothelium and scarring in the myocardium are secondary effects—effects that the cholesterol partisans have mistaken as the cause of atherosclerosis.**

The key dietary factor is not milk as such, Dr. Oster emphasizes, but the homogenization process which creates liposomes that trap the xanthine oxidase and make it biologically available. In this form, the xanthine oxidase is phagocytosed after entering the lymph stream and is released into the target tissues. **The xanthine oxidase-carrying liposomes, Dr. Oster says, are a "molecular Trojan Horse."**

In an interview with MEDICAL TRIBUNE, he summarized the epidemiologic, biochemical and preliminary clinical observations that support his hypothesis.

"Ancel Keyes, in his population studies, proved nicely that a dietary factor is responsible for the aggravation and speed of development of atherosclerosis. But his studies, and those of others fail to account for the striking differences in the incidence of coronary artery disease between populations that apparently have the same food habits. Both the French and the Finns, for example, are leading consumers of cheese and milk, but the Finns have the world's highest rates of CAD and CAD mortality. The French do not.

"In the Korean war, autopsy studies of American soldiers demonstrated a high rate of early atherosclerotic lesions but there were almost no such lesions in studies of Korean war dead of the same age."

Evidence of Homogenization's 'Bad' Chemistry?

CAD Rate Low Where Milk Is Ultrapasteurized or Boiled

By NATHAN HORWITZ
Medical Tribune Staff

"Milk is the common denominator in epidemiologic studies in the U.S. and Western Europe, and this has been the misleading aspect of all of these investigations. The assumption has been that milk is milk, everywhere the same. But the answer lies in what has been done to the milk before it is made available for human consumption. The French either boil their milk, or ultrapasteurize their homogenized milk, thereby destroying the XO. The Finns drink homogenized milk in large quantities. Similarly, the American soldiers who were autopsied in Korea had been brought up on a diet heavy with homogenized cow's milk. The Korean youngsters drank only small amounts of unprocessed milk.

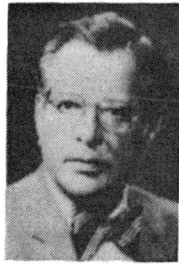

DR. OSTER

"I have been around the world twice, studying the milk-drinking habits of various peoples, and the same observation emerges repeatedly. Where bovine milk is homogenized and pasteurized, even if the intake is low, the CAD rate is high. Where the milk is merely boiled, or where cow's milk is consumed in minimal amounts, as in India, the CAD rate is low. It is not milk per se, not the milk fat, not the protein, but the xanthine oxidase, rendered bioavailable by homogenization, that creates the problem."

Dr. Oster pointed out that this concept is indirectly supported by the notably lower CAD rates in premenopausal women. "A recent hormonal study by Dr. Gregoriades Roussos of the National Institute of Dental Health, has shown that xanthine oxidase is activated by the male hormone, but inhibited by female hormones in women of child-bearing age."

Finds XO Antibodies

A major finding, and one of the important building blocks in Dr. Oster's theoretical structure of atherogenesis was his demonstration in 1974 of specific antibodies to bovine xanthine oxidase in patients with atherosclerotic disease. In a double-blind study of sera from 75 patients, Dr. Oster and his colleagues found a higher titer of XO antibodies in those with demonstrated atherosclerotic disease, whether of the coronaries or of peripheral vessels, than in those with other diseases. That study led to two conclusions: first, that exogenous XO could be absorbed and, secondly, that the test might serve as a screening procedure for the presence of atherosclerosis, without specifying an anatomic site. Investigators at the University of Delaware have since obtained corroborating results. Dr. Oster said.

"Such a test," he observed, "would be a vast improvement over the so often meaningless (because of their vast variability) serum cholesterol determinations."

Nevertheless, as noted earlier, a major stumbling block in the Oster theory has been the repeated challenge to the view that a molecule the size of xanthine oxidase (300,000 Daltons) could survive digestion in the stomach and then pass intact through the mucous membranes.

Liposomal Ploy

In their latest study, Dr. Oster and his colleague, Dr. Donald J. Ross, also of Fairfield University, believe they've answered this challenge. The strategy behind the study stemmed from a known pharmacologic phenomenon: that enzymes trapped in liposomes can be persorbed through the intestinal mucosa and that their physiologic effects are then demonstrable. "A noteworthy example of this action was the oral administration to experimental animals of liposomes carrying insulin, which subsequently effected a reduction of the subjects' blood sugar levels," Drs. Oster and Ross reported.

At the September, 1977, meeting of the New York Academy of Sciences, Drs. Oster and Ross made public a series of electron microscope photographs of XO trapped in liposomal form in homogenized cow's milk. In the same paper, they reported for the first time the demonstration of the enzyme in the cellular components of blood from volunteers after milk-loading experiments.

What do all of these findings, taken collectively, mean for the management of atherosclerosis?

"Prevention and treatment are attainable because the goal is to inhibit xanthine oxidase when indicated by the antibody test," Dr. Oster observed. "We looked for a long-term drug, without side effects, that was an XO inhibitor, and found it in folic acid. We employ it in those patients who have antibodies to XO. **Since 1970, we have used folic acid, in 20 mg tablets, in combination with ascorbic acid, q.i.d., in a study of 200 patients with atherosclerotic disease, including peripheral disease, angina pectoris, or recurrent myocardial infarction. One hundred patients serve as our controls. The average duration of treatment has been four years, with a range of four months to eight years.**

Reduced MIs

"Our preliminary findings, which we view as remarkable, show that in the treated group there has been a significant reduction of recurrent MIs, a greater relief of angina, and greater healing of leg lesions.

"In addition to its XO-inhibiting action, which affects ectopically deposited XO but not endogenous liver XO," Dr. Oster continued, "folic acid also serves as a coenzyme in the synthesis of plasmalogens. It thereby helps to repair the damage to the cell membrane brought about by the xanthine oxidase deposited from bovine milk liposomes into an unphysiologic milieu."

Dr. Oster believes the public health implications of his concept are wide-ranging. If the XO link to atherogenesis is confirmed, he emphasizes, preventive health programs would stop invoking the specter of eggs and cheese (unless the latter were made of homogenized milk) and would put an end to tampering with good cow's milk. They woul end the guilt-ridden restrictions on some of nature's tastiest and most traditional foods.

And if an affluent or overpropagandized society continued drinking the homogenized bovine product, Dr. Oster notes, an inexpensive pharmacologic remedy would be at hand in folic acid, prescribed in large doses.

XANTHINE OXIDASE AND ATHEROGENESIS
by Donald J. Ross, Ph.D.

1. Oster's theory of bovine milk xanthine oxidase induction of atherogenesis was developed over the past 30 years and was built on research reports in the world biomedical literature too extensive to review in the present report. However the theory and its gradual experimental verification can be summarized as follows:

   Plasmalogens are naturally occurring, widely distributed phospholipids which release higher fatty aldehydes when treated with mineral acids and mercuric salts. They were discovered by Feulgen in 1924 and isolated by him in 1939.
   *Feulgen, R.E., and Bersin, T. Z. *Physiol. Chem.*, 260, 217 (1939).

2. During plasmologen turnover in tissues containing it (it is a membrane phospholipid like lecithin) its aldehyde (palmitaldehyde or plasmal) can be oxidized by the bovine milk enzyme, xanthine oxidase. (XO). This was demonstrated by Oster in 1944.
   *Oster, K.A. and Mulinos, M.G., *Jour. of Pharmacology and Experimental Therapeutics*, Vol 80, 132 ff. (1944)

3. Plasmalogen is the principal phospholipid found in the cell membranes of arterial intima and myocardial tissue, not lecithin.
   *Ferrans, V.J. et al., *Jour. of Histochemistry and Cytochemistry*, Vol. 10 462 ff. (1962).

4. Plasmalogens are also present in high concentrations in skeletal muscle and the myelin of brain and nerve.
   *Thannhauser, S. J. et al., *J. Biol. Chem.*, 188, 417-427 (1951).

5. An analysis of plasmalogen-containing tissues reveals that the enzyme xanthine oxidase is lacking. Thus, XO is not found in plasmalogen-rich tissues, i.e. it is absent from cardiovascular, nervous and skeletal muscular tissue.
   *Morgan, E.J., *Biochemical Journal*, Vol 161, 1280 ff. (1926).

6. Plasmalogen was shown to be absent from infarcted myocardial tissue immediately after death and was depleted in the linings of atherosclerotic aortas as well as in aged aortas. Oster and Hope-Ross performed a histoinfarction and found that plasmalogen had disappeared from the infarcted area although there was no necrosis or other significant tissue changes of the affected heart muscle as demonstrated by routine hematoxylin-eosin staining of the same tissues. In effect, plasmalogen had leaked out of the infarcted region, *before* any other demonstrable morphologic changes had occurred.
   *Oster, K. A. and Hope-Ross, P., *Amer. Jour. of Cardiology*, Vol. 17, 1966.

7. Before this, it had been demonstrated that there is a depletion of plasmalogen in arterial tissues with age, especially in plaque areas.
   *Buddecke, E. and Anderson, G.E., *Hoppe Seiler Zeitschrift fur Physiologische Chemie*, Vol. 314, 38 ff. (1959).
   *Miller, B. et al.,

8. In view of the above, Oster postulated that the initial lesion in the arterial intima could be initiated by ectopically deposited xanthine oxidase on the intimal surface where it found a suitable substrate in the palmitaldehyde moiety of the plasmalogen in the intimal cell membranes. Since the intimal lesions can form very early in human life,

Oster surmised that the source of the ectopically deposited xanthine oxidase was dietary milk which is rich in the enzyme only 42% of which is destroyed by pasteurization.

9. More and Haust found that the coronary arteries of humans, ranging in age from the neonatal period to 25 years of age contained atherosclerotic lesions, apparently superimposed upon well developed, rather than thin intimas.
*More, R.H., and Haust, M.D., 1968. "Diffuse Intimal Thickening of Coronary Arteries in Children and Young Adults and its Role in Atherosclerosis" pp. 75-87. In: Le Role de la Paroi Arterielle dans l'atherosgenese. Colloques Internationaux du Centre National de la Recherche Scientifique. *Editions du Centre National de la Recherche Scientifique*, Paris.

10. An epidemiological investigation of the milk consumption habits of various world nations reveals that the incidence of atherosclerotic complications is significantly reduced in population groups with a high degree of lactose intolerance.
*Tejada, C. et al., 1968. Distribution of Coronary and Aortic Atherosclerosis by Geographic Location, Race and Sex. In: H.C. McGill (Ed.) *The Geographic Pathology of Atherosclerosis*. Williams & Wilkins Co., Baltimore, pp 49-66.

11. Human blood sera in ischemic heart disease contain plasmalogens in augmented concentrations, as compared with normal sera, indicating that plasmalogens are related to intimal and myocardial protection and disappear from such tissues in ischemic conditions.
*Povoa, H., et al. *Acta Biol. Med. Germ.*, Band 31, Seite 897-898, (1973).

12. Workers in my laboratory and I detected the enzyme, xanthine oxidase in atherosclerotic lesions and myocardial tissue lesions. The enzyme *was absent in normal tissues from the same patient.*
*Ross, D.J., Ptasynki, M. and Oster, K., *Proceedings of the Society for Experimental Biology and Medicine*, Vol. 144, pp. 523 ff. (1973).

13. The question arose as to the source of this misplaced xanthine oxidase. Did it come from damaged liver cells which contain the enzyme or from a dietary source, via milk and some dairy products which contain it in abundance? If from the latter source it would be possible to detect antibodies to highly purified bovine xanthine oxidase in individuals with atherosclerotic heart disease using an existing highly sensitive hemagglutination method.
*Boyden, S.J., *Jour. of Experimental Medicine*, Vol. 93 107-120, (1951).

14. A test group of 75 patient's sera revealed varying titers of specific antibodies to *bovine* xanthine oxidase. We conclude that these specific antibodies are the body's defense mechanism against a persistent ectopically deposited *bovine* xanthine oxidase.
*Oster, K.A., Oster, B., and Ross, D.J., *American Laboratory*, Vol. 6 No. 8 41-47, (1974).

15. Pasteurization of milk as is done in the United States, leaves approximately 42% of the xanthine oxidase intact and in its active state* (Greenbank, G.R. & Pallansch, M., *Jour. of Dairy Science*. Vol. 45, 958 ff. 1962). XO in milk is closely associated with the fat globule, * (Gudnason, G. & Shipe, W., *Jour. of Dairy Science*, Vol. 45, 1440 ff. (1962) and Zikakis, J. & Treece, J.M., *Jour. of Dairy Science*, Vol. 53,

644 ff., 1970). When milk is homogenized, the fat globules are reduced in size by at least 3.5 times their original dimension* (Doan, F.J., *Quart. Rev. of Pediatrics*, Vol. 8, 194 ff., 1953). As a result of this unnatural micronization, the following alterations occur to the fat globule of homogenized milk:

A. A large increase in the number of fat globules.
B. A large expansion of the fat globule surface for the absorption of xanthine oxidase.
C. As a result of 1 and 2, the biological availability of xanthine oxidase is multiplied by at least 3.5, making it that much greater than that found in non-homogenized milk.
D. This increases XO's potential for persorption through the intestinal mucosa undigested; once it passes the intestinal mucosa, it eventually reaches the bloodstream via the lymph system and is deposited ectopically by an insudative process in the heart muscle and the arterial wall.

16. The scientific and medical literature proving the absorption of large, undigested protein molecules and other equally large macromolecules and microcrystals is too extensive to review here but the literature is replete with research demonstrating the absorption of catalytically intact enzymes and their active, partially digested monomers. One paper published in 1925 reviews all of the work demonstrating the absorption of whole, undigested milk proteins back to 1844,* (Schloss, O.M.: "The Intestinal Absorption of Antigenic Protein." Harvey Lectures, Ser. 20: 156-187, 1924/25). Dr. Isselbacher of Harvard has published evidence for the absorption of undigested macromolecules by the intestines, demonstrating the absorption of the catalytically intact enzyme, peroxidase,* (Warsaw, A., Walker, W. & Isselbacher, K., *Gasteroenterology*, Vol. 66: 987-992, 1974). Davies in England had demonstrated the presence of antibodies to cow's milk proteins (not specifically to bovine xanthine oxidase as we have done) in coronary heart disease patients and found significantly higher antibody levels in those patients with coronary heart disease,* (Davies, D.F., Davies, J.R. and Richards, M.A., *Jour. of Atherosclerosis Research*, Vol. 9, 103-107 (1969) and more recently, Davies, D.F. et al. *Lancet*, 1012-1014, 1974).

17. We presented experimental evidence for the hypothesis that bovine xanthine oxidase is entrapped in liposomal form by the milk homogenization process. In this form, it will resist gastric digestion and become biologically available. This was the first demonstration of the presence of a liposome-sequestered enzyme in a widely consumed food. We concluded the results indicated that a major physical alteration by a technological manipulation of a basic food may have far-reaching biological significance.
*(Oster, K.A., Ross, D.J., Sharnick, S.V., *Proc. Soc. Exper. Bio. & Med.*, Vol. 163, No. 1, Jan. 1980).

Glossary

Angina Pectoris
: Spasmodic chest pain. Traditionally thought to be the consequence of decreased blood flow to the heart because of atherosclerotic coronary arteries.

Aorta
: The main artery carrying blood from the heart to the rest of the body.

Arrhythmia
: Any variation from the normal rhythm of the heartbeat.

Arteriogram
: X-ray photographs of the lumen of blood vessels used to diagnose occlusions of the major arteries. The blood vessels are initially injected with a radio-opaque die.

Arteriosclerosis
: Disease of the arteries affecting the media characterized by abnormal thickening and hardening. (Used interchangeably with atherosclerosis in text).

Atheroma
: Fatty degeneration or thickening of the inner wall of the larger arteries of the body.

Atherosclerosis
: A condition characterized by a hardening and thickening of the arterial wall, throughout the body, caused by the deposit of fatty materials (atheroma, q.v.) inside and outside the cells of the inner layer of the artery.

Biological Availability
: A term used to describe the ability of foods or drugs to gain access to certain tissues or organs of the body.

BMXO
: Bovine milk xanthine oxidase. An enzyme found in cow's milk and dairy products. The enzyme has been linked to atherogenesis in humans.

Coronary thrombosis
: A term used to describe a condition resulting from local damage to the lining of the coronary artery which leads to a clumping of platelets in that region. This is followed by the formation of a fixed bloodclot or thrombus which blocks the coronary artery.

Ectopic
: An adjective used to describe the abnormal positioning of a biological structure or chemical (e.g., XO) in an organ or tissue where it is normally never found.

Electrocardiogram
: A tracing of the heart's electrical activities.

Embolus
: A clot or other matter which travels through the bloodstream to lodge in a vessel and cause an obstruction of circulation.

Endogenous
: A term used to describe the generation of a chemical substance by the body itself.

Exogenous
: Term used to describe the incorporation by the body of materials synthesized outside of itself.

Endothelium
: The one-cell-thick layer of cells lining the lumen of a blood vessel.

Epidemiology
The branch of science concerned with the statistical distribution and control of a disease in a population group. Relied on heavily by followers of the hyperlipidemia and hypercholesterolemia origin of atherosclerosis in humans.

Etiology
The science concerned with establishing the cause of a disease.

Enzyme
A protein synthesized by cells which has the capacity to initiate or accelerate specific chemical reactions.

Hypercholesterolemia
A term used to describe an excessive concentration of cholesterol in the blood

Hyperlipidemia
A term used to describe the amount of lipids or fats and fatty material in the blood.

Hypertension
A condition in which blood pressure in the arteries is elevated.

Intima
The innermost layer of the arterial wall which is lined with epithelial cells.

Ischemic
A condition resulting from an inadequate supply of oxygen to cells and tissues.

Lesion
A medical term for a local injury to a tissue, e.g., the lining of an artery.

Lipid
Another word for fat.

Lumen
The channel in a blood vessel through which blood flows.

Media
The middle, muscular layer of the arterial wall; it has smooth muscle cells, elastic tissue and collagen.

Myocardial Infarction
Section of dead heart muscle tissue which has succumb to a lack of oxygen following a coronary thrombosis.

Nitroglycerine
A drug used for many years to treat angina pectoris; it usually provides rapid temporary relief of chest pain. Its mechanism of action is not clear.

Phospholipid
A term used to describe a large group of lipids containing phosphorus, exemplified by plasmalogen and lecithin. These fatty lipids are used primarily for structural purposes such as cell membranes.

Plasmalogen
A type of phosphorus-containing fatty substance similar to lecithin which is a vital component of those cell membranes found in certain tissues such as arterial, heart, or nervous tissue. Not all cells contain plasmalogen.

Plaque
A concentration of materials that accumulate on the surface of a body lining, such as blood vessel linings or surfaces.

Plasma
The fluid part of the blood.

Polyunsaturated Fats
Fats whose fatty acids contain one or more double

	bonds in the carbon chain. Generally found in plants and usually liquid at room temperature.
Propanol	A beta-blocking agent, used to treat angina pectoris and cardiac arrhythmias; a drug that blocks certain actions of the adrenal hormones.
Pulmonary	Having to do with the lungs
Renal	Having to do with the kidneys
Saturated Fats	Fats that harden at room temperature and are generally found in foods of animal origin.
Serum	The fluid part of the blood which remains after a blood clot is formed and removed; contains antibodies such as those to BMXO and a large number of other chemicals.
Serum Cholesterol	The cholesterol contained in the serum component of blood.
Thrombus	A clot in a blood vessel or in one of the heart's cavities.
Uric Acid	A compound resulting from the breakdown of nucleic acid components known as purines. High blood levels of it are often found in the disease called gout.
Xanthine oxidase	An enzyme involved in the chemical conversion of purines to uric acid in the liver. Consumption of bovine xanthine oxidase has been associated with the onset of atherosclerosis in humans.

Also available

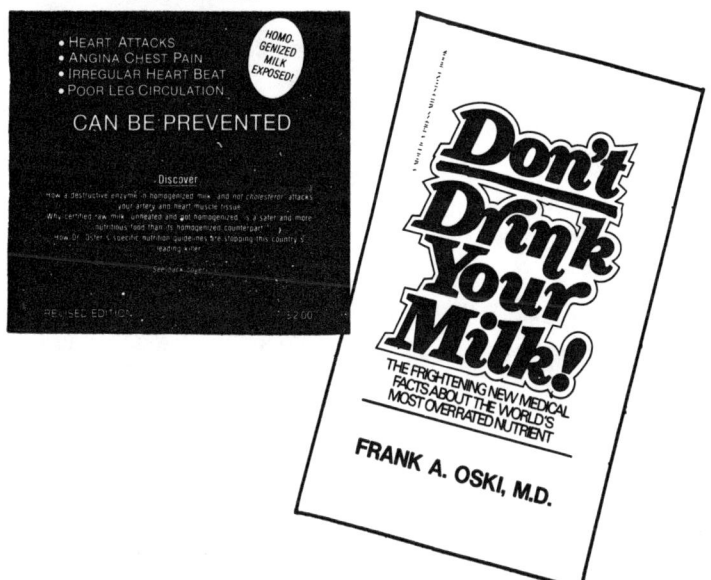